Healing Fibroids

◆ ◆

A Doctor's Guide
to a Natural Cure

Allan Warshowsky, M.D.
and Elena Oumano, Ph.D.

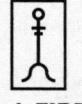

A FIRESIDE BOOK
Published by Simon & Schuster
New York London Toronto Sydney

FIRESIDE
Rockefeller Center
1230 Avenue of the Americas
New York, NY 10020

FIRESIDE and colophon are registered trademarks
of Simon & Schuster, Inc.

For information about special discounts for bulk purchases,
please contact Simon & Schuster Special Sales:
1-800-456-6798 or business@simonandschuster.com

Designed by Helene Berinsky

Manufactured in the United States of America

10

Library of Congress Cataloging-in-Publication Data
Warshowsky, Allan.
   Healing fibroids : a doctor's guide to a natural cure /
Allan Warshowsky and Elena Oumano.
     p. cm.
   Includes index.
   1. Uterine fibroids—Popular works.   2. Uterine fibroids—Treatment—
Popular works.   I. Oumano, Elena.   II. Title.
RC280.U8 W368 2002
616.99'366—dc21   2002066902

ISBN 0-7434-1824-7

CONTENTS

✦ v

INTRODUCTION

✦ Janet's Story

The bleeding came out of the blue. Janet, a woman of forty, was suddenly enduring periods so heavy that she'd go through a super-plus tampon in twenty minutes. Before long, she was bleeding between periods—then, it seemed, endlessly. Her abdomen swelled, plaguing her with a persistent, nagging pressure. Soon Janet felt constantly tired and depressed. Her regular gynecologist shrugged it off. It's not unusual for women approaching menopause to experience heavy bleeding, he told Janet. But another ob/gyn diagnosed her with a large intramural fibroid that was swelling her uterus to the size of a twelve-weeks pregnancy. He recommended a hysterectomy.

Janet's situation is typical of thousands of women across the country and many of my patients. Obviously frustrated, defenses at hair-trigger readiness, Janet arrived in my consultation room after several more gynecologists advised a hysterectomy. Janet desperately wanted to avoid surgery. She had never given birth, and she had no immediate plans for children, but she hoped, at the least, to "make it" to menopause, when reduced estrogen levels could shrink the fibroid.

Yet recent rapid and excessive growth of the fibroid had escalated the seriousness of her condition, and her doctors were urging her into the operating room because rapid growth can indicate that a fibroid is malignant.

"I don't know what to do!" a disraught Janet burst out soon after she took a seat across from me. "I still could decide to have a child someday. I also feel very strongly about not having my ovaries removed. I know their hormonal protection will keep me healthier. Plus, surgery just doesn't fit in with my plans. But for every argument I give them, my doctors throw out another counter-argument."

The Search for Answers

Just a few decades ago, "menopause," "hysterectomy," and "fibroid tumor" were hush-hush subjects that were de facto banned from the popular media. It wasn't until the early nineties—when a few ground-breaking books on the subject, like Gail Sheehy's boldly titled *Menopause,* defied centuries of silence—that information on these pressing women's health issues finally became available to the lay public. The urgent need for more and more answers remains just as strong today. You cannot open a contemporary women's magazine without reading at least one feature article on female health, and many publications have responded to reader interest by including regular columns highlighting the latest breakthroughs and discoveries in the field. Women's health issues also take up a growing share of other communications media. Two separate cable television channels, Oxygen and Lifetime, are now devoted exclusively to women's special concerns. With one-quarter of American women closing in on menopause, much of the programming on those and other channels is devoted to issues related to gynecological health. Then there's the Internet explosion. For better or worse, millions of women are now determinedly surfing the Web, hunting down the information they need to take responsibility for their health by making the right choices, including medical decisions regarding the treatment of fibroid tumors.

Fibroids and Hysterectomies

Despite the growing pool of available information, those words "fibroids" and "hysterectomy" still strike fear deep in the minds of women. And for good reason. Not long ago, a diagnosis of fibroid tumors meant a hysterectomy and the end of a woman's dream of motherhood, even her very identity as a woman. Today, modern medicine also offers procedures to shrink or remove fibroids while preserving the uterus and ovaries. But some of these procedures are questionable, and most cannot be used in the majority of cases. A staggering number of hysterectomies—half a million a year—are still being performed in this country, and the single greatest health problem that leads to this serious and life-altering operation is fibroid tumors.

For some lucky women, the condition can go completely unnoticed until discovered during a routine gynecological exam. For approximately 30 percent of white women and 50 percent of African-American women, though, these generally nonmalignant growths will cause troublesome symptoms. Fibroid tumors can be an endless source of pain, bleeding, and frustration.

Composed of fibrous muscle and tissue that grows in and around the uterus, the fibroid is among the most resistant health problems confronted by modern medicine. That is one reason why increasing numbers of women are seeking relief through alternative or holistic treatments such as nutritional therapy, herbal medicines, Chinese acupuncture, and other noninvasive, "natural" modalities. Unfortunately, the results, even with alternative natural treatments, have been mixed.

After decades of my own search for effective treatments, I can now help many of my patients heal their fibroid conditions by using a personalized treatment plan that draws on a varied arsenal of complementary treatments and strategies. These natural, holistic treatments do not conflict with modern allopathic medicine. Instead, the two schools of healing work in tandem for the patient's greater benefit.

Not only have my patients' symptoms been relieved but, in some cases, their fibroids shrank considerably. All followed individually tailored versions of a fibroid-healing program I have developed from my expanded understanding of the meaning and the means of true and complete healing.

Remember Janet? During our first appointment, Janet told her story with an attitude of frustration and hopelessness. These feelings were to play an important role in her healing. After she finished recounting her story, I asked questions about her symptoms. We then examined and evaluated Janet's diet, including any nutritional supplements she might be taking. I asked about her exercise habits, work experiences, hobbies, and meditation experience. I also wanted to know what life events, if any, could be tied to this physical problem.

Next, I performed a complete physical examination. When we returned to the consulting room, I recommended the AMAS—a test that detects malignancies in any part of the body—to rule out the possibility that her fibroid condition was malignant, because Janet's fibroid seemed to have undergone recent rapid growth. We then discussed her options. Fibroid size is evaluated in terms of different fruits—from lemon to watermelon—or various stages in a pregnancy. With a fibroid that swells the uterus to the size of a fourteen- to twenty-two-weeks pregnancy (this is the most common size I encounter), no panel of experts (called in hospitals "The Tissue Committee"), no matter how conservative, would question the decision to opt for hysterectomy.

Janet's fibroid was now twelve weeks in size. So unless the test found a malignancy, surgery was not her sole option. We went through the basic elements of the fibroid-healing program to stop growth, ameliorate symptoms, and, hopefully, shrink her fibroid. These include diet, supplements, herbs, exercise, and addressing the mental and emotional aspects of the fibroid condition. I stressed to Janet the strong commitment this program requires. In every case

I have encountered, a woman faced with the prospect of a hysterectomy will give the program six months to evaluate its effectiveness in reducing fibroid size and symptoms. After that, we reevaluate her condition and options. Janet told me she was willing to do almost anything if it could help her avoid surgery.

Her dedication paid off. Luckily, the AMAS showed Janet's fibroid was not malignant. After four months on the fibroid-healing diet and a regimen that included supplements, herbs, and other hormone-balancing substances; daily meditation/guided visualization sessions; and a brief course of psychotherapy to help her resolve issues about not having children, Janet's fibroid stopped growing and her bleeding decreased significantly. The decision whether to have a hysterectomy was no longer an issue.

Janet faithfully follows the basic principles of the program. As I write this book, five years after I met her, she remains symptom-free.

This book passes on to you the many lessons I've learned from my studies and my experiences with patients like Janet with whom I've worked from a holistic perspective on such health issues as fibroids. I did not "heal" them. We worked together on their problems by not only addressing their gynecological maladies but also taking into account their overall health, and the emotional and spiritual aspects of their healing. I wrote this book in the hope that it will provide the guidance you need to take charge of your own healing journey.

My Healing Journey

As a board-certified obstetrician-gynecologist, I have consulted with thousands of patients for more than twenty years. Yet from the first days of my practice, I came up against an undeniable truth: nothing I had learned in medical school or during my internship and residency was helping me treat a large number of my patients with any success. Many of these women came to me complaining about a complex of symptoms associated with what is known as premenstrual syndrome (PMS). Not only were they not getting better, the very concept of PMS at that time was considered a joke few doctors took seriously. Since PMS includes a vast collection of symptoms, the condition can appear to involve seemingly unrelated concerns. They include such physical symptoms as bloating, food cravings, fatigue, headaches, breast tenderness, joint pain, and pelvic congestion, as well as emotional symptoms like crying jags, aggressiveness and irritability, depression, and apathy. Premenstrual syndrome can even lead to social concerns, such as withdrawal from others and poor judgment. In my earlier years as a physician, these and other symptoms were not treated effectively because the medical establishment ignored the true and underlying diagnosis of PMS.

Frustrated by my inability to help these patients, as well as those patients suffering from endometriosis, menopausal symptoms, recurring vaginitis, and fibroid tumors, I began reading whatever I could find on new alternative and traditional natural treatments. I was desperately searching for some means to help my patients return to good health.

In an issue of *Ladies' Home Journal* back in the seventies, I came across a list of vitamins a few people were using to treat PMS with some success. I put together my own list of basics: the B complex vitamins, vitamin E, and the mineral magnesium. I also discovered that I actually helped my patients feel better simply by acknowledging the reality of their health problems and the destructive impact these had on their lives.

At the same time, I set off on a more personal journey to improve my own health. I was exploring my spirituality and experimenting with different holistic modalities—vegetarianism, meditation, yoga, and tai chi—to raise the level of my own physical and emotional condition. As my health and sense of well-being improved, I began to incorporate my discoveries into my medical practice. Soon, many of my patients were reporting that they felt better too.

Over the years, I have expanded and refined my treatment programs so that I can respond as specifically as possible to individual patient needs. This includes women who suffer from one of the most intractable of all female health complaints, fibroid tumors.

A Widespread Problem

Among women of childbearing age, the incidence of fibroids is 25 percent to 40 percent. Most of these women are in their thirties and forties, still young enough to have the families they may have postponed during their twenties, when they were busy pursuing educational degrees and establishing careers. Now their fibroid condition is jeopardizing not only their health but also their hopes for motherhood.

Here's another staggering fact: by the time they reach menopause, approximately 40 percent of American women will have a benign fibroid tumor in their uterus. Within the next ten years, 50 to 60 million American women will reach menopause. That means that over the next decade, slightly less than one-quarter of the American female population will be afflicted with this difficult, even life-threatening, condition and the hard choices it presents.

Menopause does bring with it a significant reduction in estrogen levels, and lower estrogen levels typically cause fibroids to shrink. But if these women want to go on hormone replacement therapy (HRT) to relieve menopausal symptoms and reduce the risks of heart disease and osteoporosis, their fibroids will then receive an estrogen boost that could cause them to grow. Sooner or later, too many of these women will hear from their doctors that they need a hysterectomy, and since they are no longer of childbearing age, what do they need that uterus for anyway? Sadly, hysterectomy is the second most common surgical procedure performed on women in the United States today, with each of the more than half a million hysterectomies performed annually costing, on the average, more than four thousand dollars.

Rising Interest in Alternative Medicine

There is good news! American medicine is undergoing profound changes. At least one-third of Americans now seek out alternative treatments and medicines to heal and protect their health, and 75 percent of those consumers are women. In response to this growing demand from patients, many physicians are venturing outside the confines of conventional medical training and studying such alternative or holistic modalities as acupuncture, nutrition, botanical medicine, homeopathy, exercise, and the vast and fascinating frontier popularly termed the body-mind connection.

Today, my practice is part of Beth Israel's Continuum Center for Health and Healing, in New York City. The center, which was established in 2000, is dedicated to integrating conventional and alternative schools of healing. The practitioners also include family physicians, nutritionists, an herbalist, an acupuncturist, an Ayurvedic doctor, a homeopath, a chiropractor, and other alternative practitioners. A *feng shui* master consulted on the environment so the building and its interior design would exert the most powerful healing effects possible.

Along with other groups and individual medical practitioners, the Continuum Center stands at the frontlines of a growing struggle to open up American medicine to increasingly popular complementary treatments. The new and growing discipline commonly known as complementary, integrated, or, as I prefer to call it, holistic medicine also redefines the patient from a passive body to be worked *on,* to an active partner who works *with* her doctor on her own healing.

A Holistic View of Fibroids

This book is the first to present a comprehensive yet easy-to-follow treatment plan that bridges conventional and holistic therapies. Much of the advice you will receive will enhance your health overall, because you cannot heal a fibroid condition without addressing underlying imbalances and dysfunction in your entire system. This approach is essential, because the presence of fibroids usually indicates other related, serious, even causative health problems. You will be able to use the information in this book to work on your own and to form a partnership with your doctor that will restore your health.

◆ ◆

PART ONE

THE BASICS

1

All About Fibroids

What Is a Fibroid Tumor?

No one really knows what causes fibroids, known in medical terms as leiomyomata. In fact, no one knows what causes any type of tumor at all. We do know that a fibroid is a smooth muscle tumor of the uterus that is composed of exactly the same tissue as that organ. But a fibroid is usually encapsulated by another band of tissue, and it grows independently. Many holistic health practitioners view this rogue tissue growth as nature's way of isolating and protecting the body from toxins caused by poor diet and environmental poisons that cannot be disposed of through the organs of elimination.

Practitioners of Chinese traditional medicine and other ancient Asian modalities blame blockages of "chi," or life force energy, in the channels that lead to and course through the female organs and glands. In traditional eastern medicine, the free flow of chi through these channels, also known as meridians, is the essence of optimum health.

Along with other holistic medical practitioners, I suspect that long-standing disturbances that create hormonal imbalance may be at the root of this condition. Yet all we know for sure is that the female hormone estrogen stimulates fibroid growth. Some evidence suggests that progesterone might also stimulate fibroid growth.

This theory is supported by the fact that fibroid tissue, just like uterine tissue, contains both estrogen and progesterone receptor sites. However, medical experts also know that these progesterone receptor sites may actually allow that hormone to favorably affect that tissue.

Some lucky women with fibroids have no symptoms. Others are not so fortunate. They suffer from a myriad of complaints, including lower abdominal pain and pressure, heavy menstrual bleeding, between-period bleeding, infertility, miscarriages, anemia (and associated weakness and dizziness), indigestion, chronic vaginal discharge, constipation, urinary frequency, and bladder irritation and infections.

Fibroids can grow in many different locations around and in the uterus, and there are four different types. Each type can create its own set of problems, and most fibroid conditions include at least two kinds of fibroids.

Subserous fibroids appear on the outer wall of the uterus and commonly cause the uterus to grow. This type of fibroid usually grows during menstrual periods because increased blood flow supplies it with more nutrients. Menstrual periods often cause greater abdominal bloating and worsening of all other symptoms. Subserous fibroids also typically cause painful intercourse and pain in the back and/or the groin that can even shoot down the legs. Fibroids, especially this type, can expand a uterus to the size of a watermelon or a seven-months pregnancy, which often puts pressure on adjacent organs. Pressure on the bladder or the bowels creates a whole set of problems, including constipation, incontinence, or the inability to urinate. I have even had to send some women to the emergency room in the middle of the night to be catheterized, because they were unable to urinate. This type of fibroid can cause kidney damage by pressing on the ureters, the tubes that connect the kidneys to the bladder.

Submucosal fibroid tumors develop inside the uterine cavity. They can cause severe abdominal cramping that simulates the pains

FIBROIDS (Myomata)

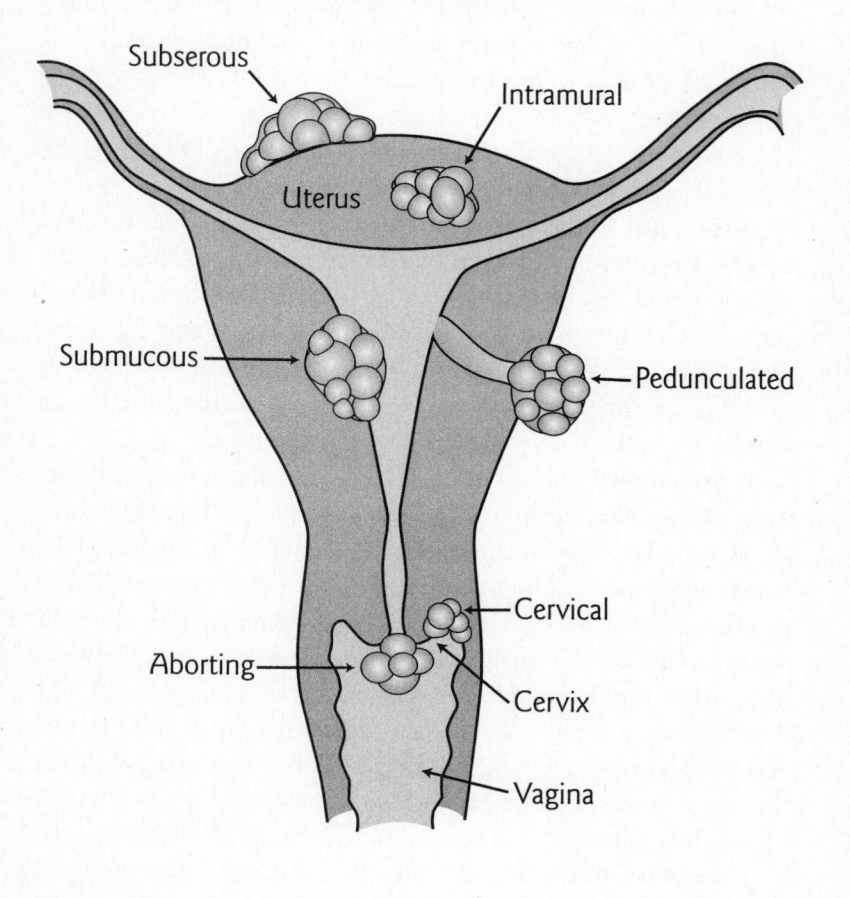

associated with childbirth, because the fibroid is situated inside the uterus, where a baby would develop. The uterus cramps because it is trying to "deliver" it, just like a baby. In a condition called "an aborting submucous myoma (fibroid tumor)," the uterus actually does expel the fibroid through the cervix and vagina, causing severe abdominal cramping and heavy bleeding. Submucosal fibroids are also typically associated with major bleeding problems. Sufferers tend to hemorrhage during heavy, often lengthy periods. Women with this type of fibroid often feel weak from blood loss. They are anemic, anxious, and frightened. In fact, submucosal fibroids bring the most women to surgery, where, all too often, they are given complete hysterectomies. Unfortunately, this type of fibroid is the most difficult to heal through holistic means.

Intramural fibroids grow within the actual uterine wall and cause many of the same symptoms as the other types. (This is the type of fibroid that brought Janet to my office.) Intramural fibroids can either grow toward the outside of the uterus and cause the same symptoms as the subserous fibroid, or grow in the direction of the inside wall, creating symptoms similar to the submucosal type.

Pedunculated fibroids are attached to the uterus by a stalk. Because of that appearance and position, they sometimes mimic ovarian tumors. This type can appear like a big ball on the outside of the uterus when imaged through ultrasound or other visual technologies. Even with modern radiological imaging techniques like CAT scans and MRIs, it is sometimes impossible to distinguish between this type of fibroid and an ovary or an ovarian cyst or tumor. For that reason, many women with pedunculated fibroids come to surgery simply to be diagnosed. If the surgeon is conservative, he or she will remove the fibroid only. But an aggressive doctor often removes the entire uterus and, sometimes, the ovaries as well. Typically, a woman with a pedunculated fibroid either feels nothing at all or, if the fibroid is pressing on another abdominal structure, she experiences cramping associated with nausea and vomiting. In cases where the pain is sharp, the pedunculated fibroid could be twisting on its stalk, causing severe abdominal pain similar to that associated with peritonitis or acute abdominal infection. Of course, this condition is a surgical emergency. As is the case with most fibroids, location is key in deciding whether or not a hysterectomy is truly indicated.

Fibroids and Cancer

Only about 1 percent of fibroids are malignant, but no one knows whether they are malignant to begin with or develop into malignancies. The only indication that a fibroid is malignant is unusually rapid growth. Even when it has been removed surgically, the pathologist must section the fibroid multiple times and count the number of cell divisions in order to detect a malignancy, because malignancy cannot be detected by the fibroid's appearance. Another way to discover whether or not a rapidly growing fibroid is malignant is by the antimalignin antibody in serum (AMAS) or AMAS test, an FDA-approved test that detects malignancy anywhere in the body. Cancer cells produce a protein called malignin. The body manufactures an antibody to malignin. If that antibody to malignin is detected by the AMAS test, we know that malignant cells are somewhere in the body. The AMAS is quite accurate, so I advise any doctor to do an AMAS test before treating a suspicious fibroid.

To Have a Hysterectomy or Not to Have a Hysterectomy?

When I was training to be a physician, if a woman over forty-five years old had any type of abdominal surgery whatsoever, the surgeon would just go ahead and remove the uterus and ovaries as well, "just in case." Today, thirty years later, the ovaries and uterus are still considered unnecessary organs after the childbearing years. Many women tell me to this day that their gynecologist said they need a hysterectomy, and since they don't plan to have more children, they "don't need" their uterus any longer. Since they are removing the uterus, the doctor might add, "Let's take out the ovaries while we're in there, so we can eliminate the possibility of ovarian cancer." When these women object that they don't want to suffer the symptoms of sudden menopause associated with this surgery, they are told, "Oh, you can take Premarin, and you'll be fine."

Too many gynecologists continue to view hysterectomy with this cavalier approach, especially when treating women over the age of forty. In cases involving larger fibroids that create serious problems, hysterectomy is necessary. Unless the fibroid condition is life threatening, though, hysterectomy should never be the first choice of treatment. Emerging evidence suggests that instead of resolving a woman's health problems, a hysterectomy can turn a bad situation worse. We now know that both the uterus and ovaries continue to perform health-enhancing functions throughout a woman's life. The ovaries produce at least four hormones *that we know of:* estrogen, progesterone, testosterone, and DHEA. The problem is that many doctors are unaware of the important role testosterone and DHEA have in maintaining hormonal balance, energy levels, and good health in a woman's later years. Testosterone is not an exclusively male hormone, as is popularly believed. Everyone needs this anabolic, or "building up," hormone to maintain and build muscle and bone and to tone the body's structure as a whole. In women, testosterone specifically works to protect the libido, promote a sense of well-being, and increase muscle tone and strength. Recent evidence indicates that testosterone is also instrumental in preventing and treating osteoporosis. A deficiency of this essential hormone has been proven to make women feel weak and fatigued; uninterested in their lives, work, and relationships; even, at times, emotionally distraught.

DHEA, popularly known as the anti-aging hormone, helps us cope with modern lives fraught with constant, heavy stress. Many busy women suffer from adrenal weakness caused by putting out too much cortisol, the hormone that is released by the adrenal glands in response to stress. This prevents the adrenals from producing enough DHEA, which leads to a deficiency. The symptoms of low DHEA levels include sleep disturbances, mood swings, and constant fatigue. Sound familiar? DHEA is also a precursor hormone, which means that your body needs it to produce other key hormones, including estrogen and testosterone. Since many of us are overstressed and therefore deficient in DHEA, we are consequently susceptible to multiple hormone deficiencies and imbalances and related health issues, such as fibroids. If a woman has a hysterectomy, she risks an even greater deficiency in DHEA.

We have learned that even the tiniest excess or deficiency of these life-sustaining natural chemicals that we call hormones can have a profoundly negative impact on our health, so you can imagine the effect on hormonal balance caused by the sudden disappearance of a woman's uterus and/or ovaries.

And that's all we know about the lifelong health-preserving functions of the ovaries and uterus so far! There may be other benefits of keeping these organs throughout a woman's lifetime that we have yet to discover.

Of course, we cannot ignore the reality that hysterectomy is a major surgery, which requires up to one year for full recovery. Nor should we ignore its possible harmful effects and complications. Not only are women of childbearing age robbed of their ability to conceive and carry a child; a significant number of women die from surgical complications. In 1975, a study found that out of 787,000 hysterectomies performed in this country, 1,700 led to the patient's death. There may be a few less hysterectomies performed these days (probably because of the influence of women's advocacy groups), but the percentage of deaths caused by complications resulting from this serious procedure is most likely the same.

Possible complications are many, varied, and sometimes severe. Many women whose uteruses are removed because of fibroids also lose their ovaries at the same time. Even if they are not removed, blood flow to the ovaries is often reduced, so that these organs no longer function well. In fact, premenopausal women who undergo a hysterectomy without ovary removal still begin menopause on the average of five years earlier than women with intact uteruses. Lowered blood flow causes their ovaries to age prematurely. Removing the uterus and ovaries causes a sudden drop in estrogen and progesterone levels, which can lead to a host of health problems that mimic the symptoms of menopause. These include vaginal dryness and sudden and severe hot flashes. Some doctors even attribute adrenal and pancreatic problems, including diabetes, to the shock of removing the female organs. Studies also indicate that for a thirty-five-year-old woman who has undergone a hysterectomy, the risk of heart attack or angina is seven times greater. Ironically, women who undergo hysterectomies to cure their fibroids are often advised after the surgery to supplement estrogen, the very same hormone that fueled the growth of their fibroids—and possibly caused other health problems—in the first place.

Most gynecologists feel that only estrogen is necessary as a hormone replacement after the uterus has been removed, despite the fact that both estrogen and progesterone receptor sites are found in many other areas of the body, such as the breasts, colon, brain, muscles, and bones. In other words, hormone balance is not just key to gynecological health, it is also essential to the body's overall health.

So why do a majority of doctors believe that a woman without a uterus needs only to take estrogen? In any case, hormone replacement therapy fails to address the underlying cause of the fibroid condition, which is hormone imbalance. In fact, hormone replacement therapy could aggravate an existing imbalance, setting up a woman for additional health problems, such as gallbladder disease, diabetes, breast disorders, and blood-clotting problems.

The list of post-hysterectomy complications goes on:

SEVERE BLEEDING. Severe bleeding can occur during the surgery and afterward. With today's concerns about the dangers of blood transfusions, bleeding has become a more significant issue.

IMPAIRED BLADDER FUNCTION. Many women suffer from post-hysterectomy bladder-function problems. They can develop a fistula, which creates a connection between the vagina and other organs. For example, if the vagina and bladder are bridged by a fistula, urine can leak into the vagina.

BOWEL INJURY. The bowels can be injured during a hysterectomy procedure.

VAGINAL VAULT PROLAPSE. During most hysterectomies, the cervix is removed, which involves cutting into the back of the vagina. This procedure sometimes leads in later years to vaginal vault prolapse, a condition in which the back of the vagina (known as the vault) falls out through the front, necessitating yet another risky surgical procedure.

LOWERED SEXUAL RESPONSE. Removing the cervix can lower a woman's sexual excitement during intercourse, because the cervix is key to sexual response in many women. In addition, many women experience the waves of orgasmic contraction and release within their uteruses. A hysterectomy robs them of that pleasure.

NEGATIVE PSYCHOLOGICAL EFFECTS. Finally, the psychological effects of a hysterectomy can be devastating. Some observers have equated hysterectomy to male castration, especially if the need for that surgery is later judged questionable. Few male physicians will accept that analogy, but the loss of a woman's womb and ovaries can be experienced as a deep psychic wound that shatters her very identity.

Despite these serious complications and outcomes, many doctors believe that the sooner and more aggresively a serious fibroid condition is addressed, the better. Medical schools do not offer their students training in holistic medicine, so many of the treatments I recommend seem to most doctors like brand-new, unproven ground. This is one reason why so many physicians are still telling their patients that hysterectomy and the newer aggressive treatments are their only options.

I wrote *Healing Fibroids* to tell you why that's just not true!

Fibroids and Hormones

Let us take a moment to sum up. You learned that no one knows all that much about why fibroid tumors develop, and few conventional doctors agree on the most effective treatments. Yet nearly all doctors—conventional and holistic practitioners alike—agree on one undeniable fact: fibroids are a serious, perhaps even escalating, threat to the health of too many American women. We have also learned that mounting evidence suggests fibroids are responsive to hormones because fibroid tissue is known to have receptor sites for both progesterone and estrogen. Other proof of the hormone connection is that women in estrogen-dominant states also tend to have large and rapidly growing fibroids. Fibroids are known to grow excessively during periods of high or excessive estrogen levels, such as pregnancy or the estrogen dominance that often occurs during perimenopause (the early stage that leads up to menopause). Once a woman is menopausal (which begins after one year of no periods) and her hormone levels become low, fibroid size often shrinks. Of course, if she is treating menopause with hormone replacement therapy, the fibroids usually do not shrink.

Some doctors try to reduce fibroid size by prescribing medications such as Synarel or Lupron to lower hormone levels; these are known as gonadotropin-releasing hormone (GnRH) agonists. But these GnRH agonists carry a risk of negative effects. One major negative effect is that GnRH agonists induce a sudden and severe menopausal state, with all the related symptoms—severe hot flashes, vaginal dryness, mood and mental changes, and increased risk for osteoporosis. Studies are being conducted on a new drug called tibolone, which is used in Europe instead of hormone replacement therapy. Tibolone is a synthetic hormone with estrogen-like and progesterone-like properties. It exerts only one-tenth the strength of the body's natural estrogen and progesterone. It can be used with GnRH agonists to reduce those negative menopausal symptoms.

Studies on the relationship between progesterone levels and fibroid growth are less than clear, because they have yielded conflicting results. Some studies suggest that high levels of progesterone reduce, even stop, fibroid growth. Other studies show just the opposite: high blood levels of progesterone lead to increased fibroid growth. One problem with these studies is that they are performed on fibroid cells in tissue cultures that are outside of the body. Studies using the anti-progesterone medication RU-486 seem to indicate that when progesterone levels are low, fibroid size reduces. But we do not know at this time what other antifibroid effects RU-486 might have. Other studies have been conducted to evaluate the effects on fibroids of the group of synthetic progesterones commonly known as progestins (Provera is one brand name). One group of women scheduled for hysterectomies took progestins for a week before surgery in order to evaluate the effect on their fibroids. After the fibroids were surgically removed, researchers noted cellular changes within the fibroids that indicated reduction in growth. All these studies and clinical results suggest to me that what really counts is not the blood level of estrogen or progesterone but the *balance* between these complementary hormones. Rather than teasing out one hormone and looking for its particular effect on fibroid growth, I believe that the balance between estrogen and progesterone and other hormones is what affects fibroid growth. Hormonal imbalance may even be a major reason why fibroids develop in the first place. Furthermore, if hormone levels are not in proper balance with each other, the presence of fibroids suggests that other imbalances—physical, emotional, and psychological—are contributing not only to the fibroid condition but also to other important health issues.

All this means that fibroids can be treated effectively, and lastingly, without resorting to invasive surgery or medications with negative side effects. It also means that a fibroid condition can become a life-enhancing opportunity. Use the advice in this book to make the necessary lifestyle changes that will improve your general health and vitality, at the same time that they relieve your symptoms by stopping, even shrinking, those fibroids.

The Real Fibroid Treatment Facts

Only a thorough evaluation of a patient's particular fibroid type and status should determine how her condition is treated. Yet studies show that those factors have less to do with a woman's treatment options—in particular, whether or not she is given a hysterectomy—than do her education level and where she lives. These studies conclude that women with only nine to eleven years of education are more likely to undergo a hysterectomy than women with higher degrees. The studies also find that certain geographical areas have a higher hysterectomy rate than other areas, particularly the South, which boasts the highest incidence of this surgery; the northeast has the lowest. In fact, areas populated by higher numbers of surgeons of all specialties show a higher rate of hysterectomies and other surgeries.

All the evidence points to the uncomfortable fact that your ability to gather information and your awareness of the options determines in large part whether or not your fibroid condition will lead to a hysterectomy. What is the lesson in this? *You must become informed so you can be in charge.*

It is true that a growing number of physicians are backing away from automatic removal of the uterus as the standard remedy for troublesome fibroid tumors. Instead, they are opting for new, more limited surgical procedures. But these options yield mixed results, limited relief, and are often associated with harmful consequences.

MYOMECTOMY. This procedure is viewed by many in the medical field as heroic because it involves removing the fibroids only and therefore should not interfere with the woman's ability to have children. Yet this surgically conservative operation is more difficult than a hysterectomy, so it must be performed by a highly skilled surgeon, and it carries the threat of negative outcomes, including excessive blood loss, infection, torn uterine lining, and perforation of the bowel. A myomectomy can also involve a rearrangement of the uterine cavity that leads to additional problems. Once the uterine cavity has been entered, any pregnancy that may follow will require a cesarean delivery because of uterine weakness caused by the surgery. Furthermore, a myomectomy, like any other pelvic surgery, can create or aggravate the hormonal imbalance that may have caused the fibroid condition. Finally, this procedure does not prevent fibroids from growing back, thereby necessitating a second operation.

CRYOMYOLYSIS. More recent fibroid-destruction techniques include cryomyolysis, in which the fibroid is destroyed by a probe-like instrument that freezes the fibroid's interior. I have performed this procedure myself under the expert guidance of a physician recommended to me because of his great success with cryomyolysis. I performed the technique several times under his supervision and have yet to see a successful outcome, either with my own patients or other women who have undergone the procedure and then consulted me. One patient even had to return to surgery a few days later because of intra-abdominal bleeding and extreme pain.

ELECTROMYOLYSIS. Electromyolysis also destroys the fibroid's interior by using a probe; in this case, by passing an electrical current through it. Again, this is a relatively new, experimental method that may or may not be successful and usually only in certain situations.

LASER MYOLYSIS. This is another addition to the various procedures for "pithing" the fibroid and destroying its interior with some sort of energy force. Laser myolysis uses laser beams. All these myolysis procedures effectively relieve fibroid growth but, at best, only for the short term. At worst, they create more problems.

UTERINE ARTERY EMBOLIZATION. Embolization is a procedure that has been used successfully in the past to reduce severe uterine bleeding during an operation. Recently it has been adapted to treat fibroids. The technique involves passing inert substances through blood vessels in the leg that lead into the pelvic area, so these vessels that nourish the fibroids are blocked. Blood flow to the fibroid decreases, causing it to shrink. But embolization techniques do not always work, and because no long-term follow-up is yet available on this relatively new procedure, we do not know how long its effects last or what the negative effects could be. In addition, embolization techniques are performed by a new medical specialty, interventional radiologists. Since many of these physicians use their own criteria to select candidates for the procedure, it is likely that embolization techniques cannot be used to treat the majority of fibroid conditions.

HYSTEROSCOPY. Some doctors are opting for hysteroscopy to treat submucosal fibroids. The surgeon guides a resectoscope, a wand-like instrument linked to a video monitor and ending in a surgical "loop," through the vagina into the uterus, where the resectoscope "shaves" the fibroid from the uterine wall. Although this option seems less aggressive than a hysterectomy, it is not a benign procedure. Large volumes of fluid need to be instilled into the uterus in order to visualize the fibroid, and problems with fluid absorption are common. Women have actually died from fluid imbalances caused by this procedure.

SUPRA-CERVICAL HYSTERECTOMY. A supra-cervical hysterectomy removes only the portion of the uterus containing the fibroids, leaving the rest of the organ intact. This procedure does not preserve fertility, but it does leave most of the pelvic support structure intact, which reduces risk of bladder-function impairment and other hysterectomy-linked complications, such as vaginal vault prolapse.

Again, none of these procedures ensures that the fibroids will not reappear or regrow, and none is effective for all fibroid conditions. *Even more important, none of these surgical options deals with correcting the underlying health problems that created the fibroids in the first place.*

The picture I have painted so far may seem to predict a grim future for the nearly half of all American women who will be diagnosed with fibroids in their lifetime. But it's not a complete picture. Much more can be done to heal a fibroid condition than removing the ovaries and uterus or even cutting, slicing, burning, or freezing fibroids out of a woman's body.

When used correctly, natural holistic healing modalities offer practical and effective solutions for healing many women's chronic health problems, including fibroids. Thankfully, increasing numbers of committed health-care practitioners and their patients are exploring these options.

These days, my practice is truly complementary, blending conventional gynecological modalities with a holistic approach to women's health.

✦ Ann's Story

Ann, like many of my patients, came to me soon after her doctor recommended surgery, in her case, a myomectomy, for her fibroid condition. A thirty-seven-year-old kindergarten teacher, Ann had recently married and was eager to start a family. Large intramural fibroids had blown up her uterus to the size of a ten-weeks pregnancy, rendering the prospect of children nearly impossible. Because Ann also suffered from irregular periods, a symptom commonly associated with submucosal fibroids, I suspected that at least some of her fibroids were of the submucosal type. This would mean that her condition was more serious, because submucosal fibroids compete with a fetus for space. Ann's regular gynecologist had recommended a myomectomy before she became pregnant, because fibroids typically grow during the hormone-enriched state of pregnancy, and they can even be associated with miscarriage. Ann was caught between her fear that the fibroids would grow during pregnancy and the possibility that even after this difficult procedure, they would return. Then there was the chance that during surgery, the physician might decide she needed a hysterectomy after all. While Ann was weighing her options, a friend recommended that she consult me to explore the possibility of alternative treatment solutions.

During the history-taking session, I learned that Ann had been a sickly child who had taken many courses of antibiotics for ear infections, sinus problems, sore throats, and other ailments.

Throughout her adult life, she had experienced many vaginal yeast infections. Ann reported to me that she had normal bowel movements. But as we continued to talk about her health status, I realized that Ann's notion of "normal" bowel movements was twice a week. My physical examination showed that Ann indeed had ten-weeks-size fibroids, but I also discovered that she did not have the submucosal type that might have necessitated surgery before she conceived.

It was clear that Ann suffered from digestive and absorption problems. Among these was a microbial imbalance in her digestive tract: too little beneficial bacteria coupled with an overgrowth of yeast. This was probably causing her constipation. In such cases, the woman invariably has increased levels of the enzyme beta-glucuronidase. Beta-glucuronidase "unpackages" estrogens that have been "packaged" for excretion. In other words, the estrogens that Ann should have been eliminating through bowel movements were being taken out and put back into circulation. This was worsening the estrogen-progesterone imbalance that was at least partially responsible for her fibroid growth.

One of the many ways in which the fibroid-healing diet arrests fibroid growth is by improving digestion, absorption, and elimination. It does this by restoring proper bacterial balance in the gut.

I test for a healthy intestinal environment with a special functional stool test called the Comprehensive Digestive Stool Analysis, by the lab Great Smokies. This test analyzes parameters of digestion, absorption, beneficial bacteria and potentially pathogenic gut bacteria, and yeast overgrowth, and it evaluates for the presence of parasites that can create symptoms of chronic illness. The test also determines the level of the specific metabolic markers that indicate a healthy intestinal environment. These markers include intestinal acidity or pH; the presence of healthy fatty acids, such as butyric acid, which is used as fuel for intestinal cells; and the presence of the enzyme beta-glucuronidase. The wrong levels of these markers suggest intestinal dysbiosis, which is a measure of disease in the digestive tract that can affect hormonal balance.

For example, beta-glucuronidase is produced by "bad" gut bacteria. It disrupts the bond between estrogen and the glucuronic acid molecule that helps escort estrogen out of the body. When this happens, the estrogen that was meant to be eliminated returns instead to the body's pool of estrogen. The result is an increase in that body's estrogen-dominant state. So beta-glucuronidase levels can be brought back to normal by correcting the imbalance in the intestinal bacterial environment. Until intestinal balance is restored, I use the nutritional supplement calcium-D-glucarate to reduce the levels of beta-glucuronidase. It is very effective in reducing this enzyme at amounts of 500 to 1,000 mg per day. There are no known negative effects and no negative side effects.

Intestinal yeast overgrowth can also increase estrogen levels by producing a toxin that mimics estrogenic effects. To correct yeast overgrowth, I use an intestinal restorative program called the 4-R Program—Remove, Restore, Reinoculate, and Repair—designed by Dr. Jeffrey Bland. This program removes abnormal irritants like bacteria, yeasts, parasites, and food allergens; then replaces stomach acid, enzymes, bile salts, and fiber; then reinoculates the intestines with healthy intestinal bacteria like acidophilus and bifidobacter; and finally repairs the intestinal walls with nutrients like glutamine, inulin, zinc, and vitamin B_5. The program takes about four to six weeks to complete, and I have found it extremely successful in dealing with intestinal dysbiosis and in helping to restore estrogen balance. A healthy digestive tract easily removes excess estrogen from the body, thereby helping hormone levels return to a healthy balance. Other elements in Ann's fibroid-healing program included various herbs, supplements, and other remedies to reduce harmful enzyme levels and restore hormonal balance. In addition, Ann practiced relaxation and visualization exercises that included "seeing a healthy baby growing in my uterus." In fact, Ann and her husband did this latter exercise together, which strengthened their relationship and made them feel like genuine partners in her subsequent pregnancy. Ann's story had a happy ending. Her fibroids stopped growing almost immediately after she started the program, and, within a few months, she was pregnant. Nine months later, she delivered a health baby girl. Ann is sticking to her fibroid-healing lifestyle to ensure her dream of a large family.

In addition to the five basic elements of the fibroid-healing program—diet, supplements, herbs, exercise, and mind/spirit work—I also recommend other holistic modalities, whenever appropriate. These include acupuncture, acupressure, other herbal traditions like Ayurvedic and traditional Chinese medicine, and homeopathy. Some of my patients feel very strongly about particular ethnic healing traditions or other arcane therapies, and I support their individual needs and beliefs. This fosters a true partnership between us and helps them create a healing environment. The most important point about the entire program is to allow the complementary actions of the various healing systems that you have put into practice to awaken your own inner healer.

The fibroid-healing program is comprehensive and inclusive, and it demands commitment, but when a woman approaches her healing with that profound level of dedication, "miracles" do happen.

Healing Fibroids can guide and support your own miracle. Use the information and direction I provide in this book to develop a healthier lifestyle and make informed health decisions, either with your health-care practitioner or on your own. The program will guide you to a way of living that will help relieve your symptoms and arrest fibroid growth by restoring your body to optimal health and balance. If you do not suffer from fibroids, the fibroid-healing program will help prevent them by ensuring optimal health.

In my medical practice, I take many possible factors into account whenever I assess a patient's unique situation. Each of the following chapters helps you evaluate your own situation by taking you through a key component of the fibroid-healing program. You will reexamine each aspect of your lifestyle and learn where you could make positive changes to maximize your health and promote your own healing. You will take a good, hard look at your diet and its relationship to the digestive and hormonal problems linked to fibroid conditions. You will learn about nutritional supplements and herbs that boost gynecological health and hormone balance. You will discover the benefits of various types of exercise to fibroid conditions. You will learn effective, fun ways to reduce and relieve the effects of stress. You will learn how to relieve the burden of any psycho-emotional factors that may be responsible, at least in part, for creating your fibroid condition. These include possible unresolved issues relating to your sexuality, relationships, gender identity, creativity, or past traumas. You will also be given suggestions on how to resolve these issues so that they no longer compromise your health. Finally, you will learn how to create a daily meditation and guided visualization practice that will help you heal on every level of your being.

2

The Hormonal Web, the Menstrual Cycle, and Fibroids

The Hormonal Web

Science may not fully understand why fibroids develop and grow, but we know that fibroid development and growth are linked somehow to the body's hormone system. Holistic physicians take a broader, more profound view of the relationship between fibroid tumors and the hormone system. They see a connection between the development and growth of fibroid tumors with an ongoing, organic, and all-inclusive body process known as the hormonal web. The hormonal web ties together your body's psycho-neuro-endocrine-immune systems. The interconnections within this vast complex of body-mind systems are as intricate and as exquisitely delicate as a spider's web.

Your menstrual cycle also connects to, and affects, virtually every aspect of this complicated hormonal web. When each of the many elements included in the web does its part to maintain health and balance in your body, it is as if it were an instrument in a huge and splendid orchestra. But when even just a few players fall out of sync with the others, the result is no longer beautiful music but chaos. That is, irregularities in your body's hormone balance and menstrual cycles leave you vulnerable to fibroid development and growth, as well as to other gynecological dysfunction.

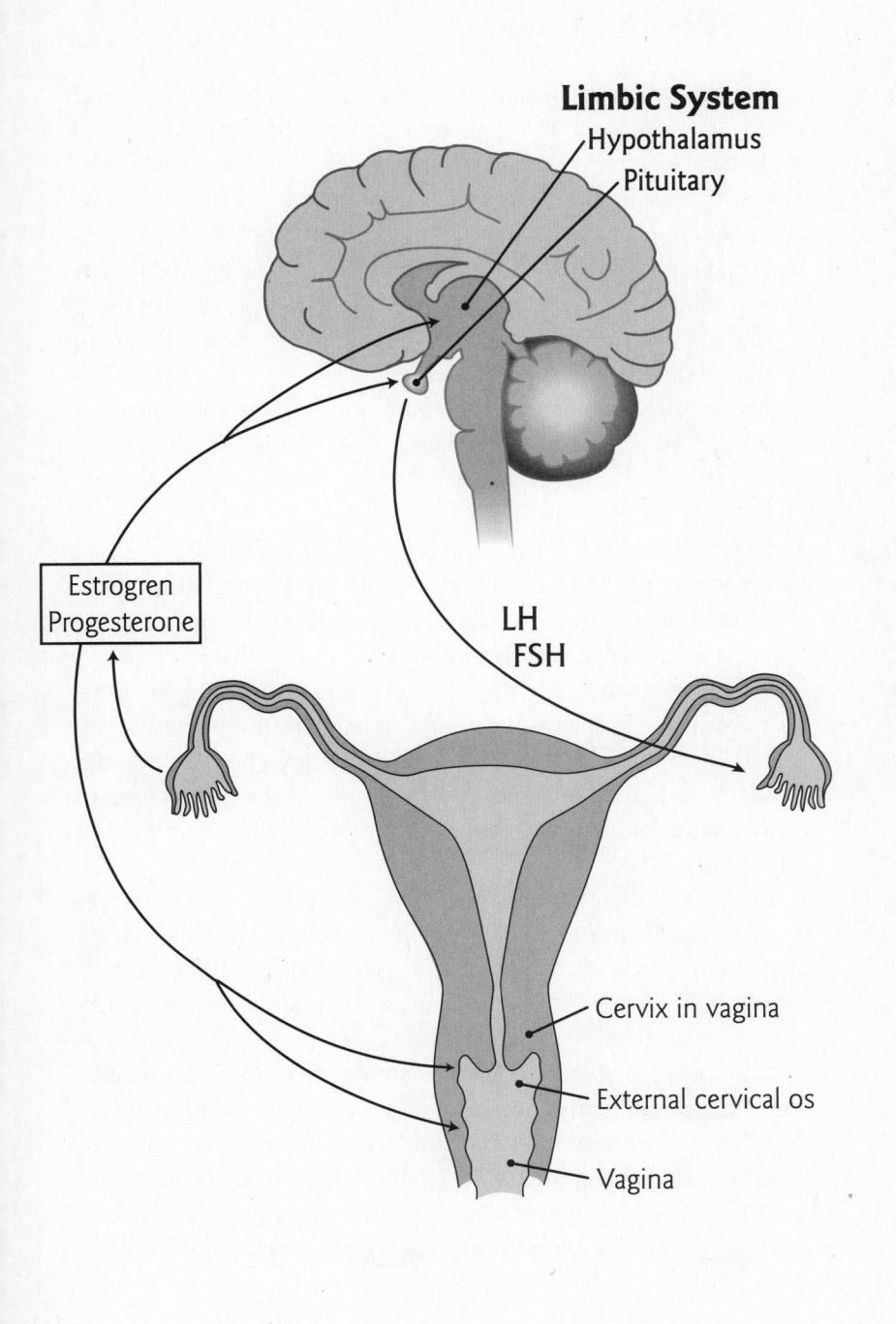

Limbic System
Hypothalamus
Pituitary

Estrogren
Progesterone

LH
FSH

Cervix in vagina

External cervical os

Vagina

The hormonal web requires balance among body, mind, and spirit. The need for a healthy body, mind, and spirit is particularly important when it comes to the phases of your menstrual cycle. Here's why. Each phase of the menstrual cycle is "cued" by various components of your hormone system. That hormone system is breathtakingly sensitive and easily thrown off balance. Any disruption in the hormone system, no matter how subtle, can lead to a myriad of gynecological complaints, from PMS to endometriosis to the development of fibroid tumors.

Let us take a look at the various components of the hormonal web and how its chain of signals regulates your menstrual cycle.

THE HORMONE SYSTEM

HYPOTHALAMUS GLAND. The hypothalamus gland is our first player in the hormonal symphony. It "sits" in the midbrain, under the limbic area, where it receives signals from the limbic brain telling it when to release hormones. Once the hypothalamus gets its instructions, it sends its own hormonal signals down to the pituitary gland, also known as the master gland of the hormonal system.

PITUITARY GLAND. After being cued by the hypothalamus, the pituitary gland then relays its own messages to other key players in the hormonal system: the ovaries, the adrenal glands, and the thyroid gland.

Within this chain of signals, each player is stimulated to secrete its own specific hormone, or group of hormones, in order to create changes in corresponding parts of the body. Each hormone stimulates its own specific target areas in the brain and the rest of the nervous system, where neuropeptides are created.

NEUROPEPTIDES. Neuropeptides are the messengers of the nervous system; they carry impulses everywhere in the body.

OVARIAN HORMONES. Ovarian hormones include estrogen, progesterone, testosterone, and DHEA. These ovarian hormones stimulate a response that ensures that the rest of the body—including lungs, heart and blood vessels, and bone—functions normally.

Ovarian hormones exert a powerful effect in the breasts, an area of great concern to women, because studies link hormonal imbalance to the possible stimulation of cancer. On the other hand, balanced hormone function helps maintain normal changes in the breast tissue. For example, balanced hormone function helps the breast change so that a newborn can be nourished with breast milk.

Hormones affect your entire genital area—the vagina, the bladder, and the lower gastrointestinal tract. Nowhere else is the ebb and flow of a smooth hormonal concert more evident than in the uterus. In women of childbearing age, the uterus prepares itself for the possibility of a fertilized egg through the continual buildup and breakdown of the uterine lining (also known as the endometrium). If conception does not occur, that lining is shed as a monthly menstruation.

Hormones cooperate in the continuous remodeling of your bones' architecture. They help repair microscopic cracks and breaks in an effort to maintain the integrity of this vital and dynamic body system. Hormones also drive repairs of your skin and muscle.

In fact, the endocrine glands, the hormones they secrete, and the brain's neuropeptides work together on the continuous repair and remodeling process that helps maintain optimal function of virtually every part of your body.

HORMONE RECEPTOR SITES. Hormones are able to do their essential work because all body areas contain appropriate hormone receptor sites on the membranes that line each and every cell. The process is nothing short of miraculous. Each cell's receptor site is precision-designed to fit only the right hormone, in much the same way a key is precision-fit to a specific lock, or a docking area is designed to receive a specific ship.

Imagine each hormone molecule as it travels through the bloodstream, sailing through the blood vessels until, like an oceangoing cruise ship, it arrives at its "dock"—its particular hormone receptor site. Imagine a huge vessel like the *Queen Elizabeth 2* trying to squeeze itself into a dock designed for a submarine. In the same way, a hormone cannot connect with just any receptor site to do its work. The hormone must be specific for that site. Yet, once the right hormone successfully "docks" in its receptor site located on a cell's membrane, it is smoothly escorted through that membrane into the cell's interior. That interior is called the cytoplasm, and it contains the nucleus, or command center of the cell.

HORMONE-RECEPTOR COMPLEX. The cell nucleus is also surrounded by a membrane, which means that the hormone must pass through this second membrane via another specific hormone site or dock. Once it gets through and enters the cytoplasm, a hormone-receptor complex is created. The hormone-receptor complex is what does the work by creating a protein messenger that will set off certain events in that part of the body.

I use the term "hormone-receptor complex" to describe the point at which hormones and their receptor sites interreact, because scientists now believe that when the hormone and its receptor site combine, they form a third and new structure. The new structure is different from either the hormone or its receptor site, and it is this new structure that actually creates protein messengers that create necessary changes in your body.

For example, bone contains receptor sites for both estrogen and progesterone. When the progesterone-receptor complex forms in a bone cell's nucleus, it stimulates that bone cell to produce a protein messenger molecule that actives the osteoblast. The osteoblast is a specific cell whose job is to lay down new bone wherever repairs are needed. The need for bone repair can result from something as minor as bumping your funny bone, which sets off that strange, electric buzz in your elbow. Or the job can be as major as a severe fracture of the hip, where old bone first must be removed in order for new bone to be laid down. But the body cannot build new bone unless the complex action of the hormone progesterone and its receptor site cause the messenger molecule to notify the osteoblast that it is time to start building. At the same time that the progesterone-receptor-site complex signals the osteoblast to lay down new bone, the estrogen-receptor-site complex in bone tissue does its own complementary work: making sure that old or damaged bone is removed by bone-removing cells called osteoclasts.

This elaborate hormonal dance to maintain healthy bone structure is just a single instance of complex interactions between hormones and their receptor sites that keep your entire body in optimal balance and health.

DISRUPTIONS IN THE HORMONE SYSTEM

Any number of problems can appear at any time to disrupt this extremely fine-tuned system. If the nuclear membrane of a cell is healthy, the appropriate hormone molecule can easily maneuver itself into the command center. But if either the outer membrane or nuclear membrane is not healthy, the hormone will not be able to get inside and do its work. As you will learn in detail a bit later in this chapter, the health of cellular membranes and nuclear membranes can be compromised by poor lifestyle choices. These include an unhealthy diet, lack of exercise, too little rest, and the inability to cope with stress. If enough hormones cannot enter cells, key body processes will be disrupted, and you become vulnerable to a wide spectrum of disorders associated with hormonal imbalance, including the development and growth of fibroid tumors.

The good news is that all it takes to restore the health of these hormone receptor sites are simple changes in your lifestyle.

XENOESTROGENS. Xenoestrogens are not part of the hormonal web, but they are the pretenders that masquerade as hormones. This group of chemicals includes pesticides and insecticides (such as DDT, DDE, and dieldrin), organic solvents, PCBs (polychlorinated biphenyls), and plastics. Xenoestrogens are everywhere in our modern lives, and once their molecules enter the body, they trick it so they can dock in hormone receptor sites designed for our natural hormones. They are modern villains that act as foreign estrogens whenever they get into the body. For that reason, they are another major disrupter of the precision balance that involves hormonal secretions, hormone receptor sites, receptor-site activation, and hormone-receptor complexes. Your body's natural hormones may not be doing their job because xenoestrogens are beating them to their receptor sites and exerting negative, hormonelike effects on your body. By mimicking the action of hormones without creating the desired results, xenoestrogens can cause either no body response, exaggerated responses, or altered responses. Once they enter a cell via hormone-receptor-site complexes, they can set off abnormal cellular responses that can have devastating consequences for your health. Studies prove that xenoestrogens have already wreaked havoc in the animal kingdom. They are causing widespread infertility and many other reproductive problems, as well as other abnormalities in creatures that inhabit marshes and waters that have been polluted by runoff from pesticides and insecticides. Bird and reptile eggs show abnormalities ranging from extremely thin and fragile shells to failure to hatch, and animals show gender irregularities. For example, alligators in the Florida Everglades are exhibiting extremely low testosterone levels and abnormally small penises.

It does not take a great leap of logic to realize that xenoestrogens are causing the same reproductive and health problems among humans. Male sexual function also depends on a similarly intricate and sensitive process to create hormone-receptor-site complexes. During my more than twenty years of medical practice, I have witnessed the normal sperm count for men drop from a minimum of 60 million sperm per cubic centimeter of ejaculate to about 20 million. Probably the most dramatic example of the effect xenoestrogens have on the human symphony of hormonal interactions involves the story of the drug diethylstilbestrol.

Diethylstilbestrol (DES) is a synthetic estrogen that was used in the fifties and sixties to prevent miscarriage. Ironically, the drug not only proved ineffective for that purpose, it also caused irreversible and devastating changes in human reproductive tissue. The female offspring of women who received DES were found in later life to show an increased incidence of a rare form of vaginal cancer, called adenocarcinoma. DES's adverse effects may never have been discovered if this type of cancer were not otherwise so rare. Other changes developed in the vaginal and cervical tissues of DES daughters that required constant medical surveillance through Pap smears and microscopic examinations of the cervix called colposcopies. Cervical and vaginal biopsies may also have to be performed on these daughters, in order to rule out malignant changes in these tissues. Researchers are currently discovering that the male offspring of women who took DES also show changes in their reproductive organs. Ongoing studies on the second-generation offspring—the grandchildren of DES mothers—are being conducted to determine whether or not they will also suffer the negative effects of this dangerous xenoestrogen.

Xenoestrogens can also disrupt the normal chain of hormonally driven events in an opposite manner, by making a receptor site resistant to its appropriate hormone, so the necessary hormone-receptor-site complex cannot be created. Xenoestrogens and other factors can disrupt normal hormone-receptor-site action so easily that I am at times amazed whenever *any* body process takes place normally. Yet our bodies usually do perform as they should! One of the hormonal web's most awesome feats is regulating a woman's monthly menstrual cycle. Let us take a look at what happens in a typical cycle.

THE MENSTRUAL CYCLE

DAY ONE. Day 1 of a normal menstrual cycle is marked by the onset of the menstrual flow. At this phase of the cycle, estrogen and progesterone levels are at their lowest, monitored by a feedback system that continually checks hormone levels in the bloodstream. On day 1, the pituitary gland perceives that blood levels of estrogen are low, so that gland increases its production of follicle-stimulating hormone (FSH). The pituitary gland is "helped" in this job by the hypothalamus, which stimulates the pituitary by releasing its own

Menses cycle

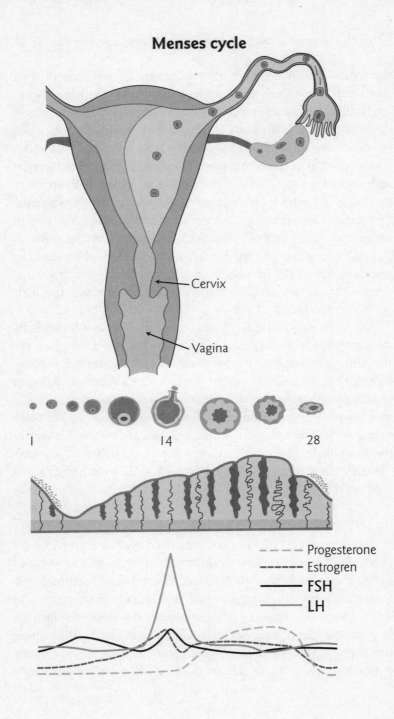

Cervix

Vagina

1   14   28

Progesterone
Estrogren
FSH
LH

hormone, GnRH. Of course, the hypothalamus is acting, in turn, under orders from the brain's limbic system. (We will get more into this fascinating system and its relationship to fibroids and gynecological health a little later on. For now, let us continue tracking the phases of a normal menstrual cycle.)

After the hypothalamus has stimulated the pituitary gland to increase FSH production in response to low estrogen blood levels, the FSH stimulates specialized cells within the ovarian follicle to produce more estrogen. Actually, the term "estrogen" is somewhat misleading. At this stage, we really are talking about stimulating the production of three different human hormones that are grouped together as "estrogens." They are:

Estradiol. The principal estrogen is called estradiol, or E2. This is the most abundant estrogen present during the so-called reproductive years. (Of course, women are productive throughout their lives!)

Estrone. Estrone, or E1, is usually interchangeable with estradiol and is equally strong. Estrone is ordinarily the most abundant estrogen during menopausal years and has been implicated in breast cancer formation. During menopause, testosterone precursor molecules called androstenedione, which are found in fat cells, are converted into estrone. This conversion is a double-edged sword. On one hand, a little extra fat can reduce the uncomfortable symptoms of menopause and ease various menopause-related health problems. For example, extra fat lowers the risk of osteoporosis. On the other hand, too much fat can increase estrone levels, thereby creating a higher risk of estrogen-dependent problems, such as breast cancer and gallbladder disease. Of course, the risk for these diseases is even greater with poor lifestyle choices, such as a bad diet.

Estriol. The third estrogen, estriol, is the weakest of the estrogens that occur naturally in human beings. Estriol is most abundant during pregnancy, and it appears to be a biological end product of the two stronger estrogens. In some studies, estriol has been found to protect against breast cancer. In an article that appeared in the *Journal of the American Medical Association* (*JAMA*), Dr. Alvin Follingstad called estriol "the forgotten estrogen," and wrote about a discovery made during the seventies by Dr. Henry Lemon, called "The Estrogen Quotient." Lemon measured the amounts of each of the three estrogens in the urine of premenopausal women. He found that the women with higher amounts of estriol showed the least incidence of breast cancer. Lemon discovered that when a woman had sufficient estriol in her twenty-four-hour urine collection—that is, when the total amount of estriol divided by the sum of estradiol and estrone was greater than 1.7—she experienced a lowered risk of breast cancer. This discovery suggests the possible protective role of estriol against breast cancer. No one has followed up with studies to confirm or disprove Dr. Lemon's conclusions, but it seems like a good idea to keep your estriol levels high as you go through menopause. You will learn in later chapters how to do this easily through simple changes in your diet and improvements in your lifestyle.

DAY TWO. The special cells in the ovaries that are stimulated to produce more estrogen through the action of the FSH sent by the pituitary are called theca cells. As the theca cells continue to mature, they produce more and more estrogen. As levels of estrogen in the bloodstream rise, all the early warning signs and symptoms of the menstrual cycle are set off. One of those signs is an increase in the mucus secreted by the cervix. (The cervix is the opening to the uterus located at the back of the vagina. See the illustration on page 40.) Estrogen also causes that mucus to become more sticky and stretchable. If you place a small amount of this cervical mucus between two fingers and then stretch them apart, the mucus will stretch as well, without breaking. This quality is called the "Spinbarkeit effect," and it is used in family planning as a way to detect the hormonal changes that occur just before and during ovulation.

MIDPOINT. As the menstrual cycle approaches its midpoint, estrogen levels continue to rise. For most women, this happens on about day 14, but it can actually occur anywhere from day 3 to day 21 within a normal cycle. At that midpoint, via a mechanism that is still not completely understood, the pituitary gland releases a specific, pulsed amount of luteinizing hormone, also known as LH. During this phase, the ovary is still under the effect of continued FSH stimulation, and several ovarian follicles—each containing a premature egg—are developing. Every woman is born with approximately 1 million immature eggs in her ovaries. As the time for that midcycle pulse of LH approaches, one follicle identifies itself as the one that will release its egg that month, and the other follicles regress. In effect, they back away, almost as if they were sacrificing themselves, and regressed follicles are not likely to be stimulated ever again.

At this point in the cycle, the "victorious" follicle is still under the direction of LH, which we can call the "hormone of the moment." The LH causes the follicle to release its egg, also known as the ovum, into the abdominal cavity. Here is where we enter the realm of the truly amazing. That tiny, microscopic-sized egg is simply expelled, helter-skelter, into the abdominal cavity. It could land anywhere in the depths of this intensely crowded and hyperactive part of the body. Yet the egg, also known as the ovum, is detected and rescued from oblivion by the fimbria, the fingerlike projections at the ends of the fallopian tubes (see the illustration on page 40). The fimbria of one fallopian tube pick up the egg through another mechanism that remains one of medical science's most intractable mysteries.

After it has been caught up by those fingerlike projections, the egg travels down the length of the fallopian tube. Again, no one really knows just how this is accomplished. We do know, though, that whenever effective transport of the egg is delayed for any reason, the chance greatly increases for an ectopic, or tubal, pregnancy. If the fimbria fail to grasp the egg so that it drops deep into the abdominal cavity, other problems can result. If the egg is not fertilized by sperm, it is no big deal. But if egg fertilization does take place, a rare but dangerous pregnancy can occur, in which the developing fetus attaches to the intestinal wall and creates an abdominal pregnancy with potentially devastating effects on both mother and fetus.

Normally, fertilization takes place within the fallopian tube. Just to make this fascinating tale even more astounding, consider what can happen in women having only one fallopian tube because the other one was removed surgically. The remaining fallopian tube can reach all the way across the abdominal cavity to grab the egg as it emerges from the ovary on the other side of the body, thereby setting the stage for a successful pregnancy!

The body's ability to pull off such magnificent feats has taught me never to take anything about human health for granted and always to expect the unexpected.

To continue our account of the menstrual cycle, let us see what happens after the egg is picked up by the fallopian tube. The empty follicular sac in the ovary does not just turn into waste. It converts itself into a progesterone-secreting organ that is called the corpus luteum. Nature in all her wisdom uses everything at her disposal, and this particular transformation makes the most effective use possible of the empty, semi-destroyed follicle, or egg sac.

The corpus luteum, what was formerly just an empty egg sac, now produces progesterone in order to balance the effect of estrogen in the uterus, so that the uterus is prepared to accept and nurture the fertilized egg.

This ideal balance of progesterone and estrogen in the uterus allows a fetus to develop and become a child. A balance between progesterone and estrogen is equally necessary to maintain the health of other hormonally responsive body parts, such as the breasts, bone, heart, and brain.

THE SECOND PHASE. Estrogen primed the uterus during the first part of the cycle to build up its lining, or endometrium. During the second half of the cycle, the rise in progesterone causes the uterine lining to stop growing. Progesterone also stimulates the endometrial cells to differentiate so they can create the proper environment for nurturing a fertilized egg. It does this until approximately the twelfth week of pregnancy, when the placenta has developed enough to take over that job. If there is no pregnancy, the corpus luteum—formerly known as the destroyed follicle casing—produces progesterone for approximately two weeks of a cycle.

When the corpus luteum stops functioning after two weeks, it becomes the corpus albicans. This second transformation causes progesterone levels to plummet. Lowered progesterone levels are the signal for the built-up uterine lining to be sloughed off as the menstrual flow. Menstrual flow usually occurs on day 28 of the cycle, but many women experience a normal cycle that is substantially shorter or longer. Of course, once the flow ends, we are back to day 1, and the entire menstrual cycle repeats itself once again.

Other major players in this wonderful concert are the pituitary gland, which includes in its job description stimulating the adrenal glands, and the thyroid gland, which also produces and secretes adrenocorticotropic hormone (ACTH) and thryoid-stimulating hormone (TSH). All these hormones are important to your overall health, and they are also key to your menstrual cycle and other gynecological functions, because they are essential for a healthy balance between estrogen and progesterone secretions.

As I have mentioned already, hormone balance and menstrual cycles can be disturbed by extremely subtle influences, some of which are still unknown to medical science. For example, a well-known phenomenon confirmed by many studies occurs whenever a group of women live together, such as in a college dormitory. In these instances, a "dominant" female will control the menses of the other girls. Initially, the "follower" women feel as if they are experiencing irregular periods. Eventually, they realize that all their cycles have come to coincide. As soon as my daughter began her menses, my wife's periods and my daughter's seemed to tune in to each other. After just a few months, their periods were almost completely synchronized. One theory explains this phenomenon through pheromone production. The "dominant" female is the one who produces the most powerful pheromones. Pheromones are chemical entities that stimulate the olfactory nerves in the brain, enabling you to detect smells. These pheromones also stimulate the brain's limbic system, the hypothalamus, and the pituitary—all which, as you now know, play key roles in controlling the phases of the menstrual cycle.

A regular menstrual cycle depends on such precise interplay between several glands and such tiny amounts of hormonal secretions that they are measured in units known as picograms, a trillionth of a gram, and nanograms, a billionth of a gram. Any disturbance in the balance between hormone levels, even at the nanogram or picogram level, can severely disrupt a woman's health and create a host of problems, including fibroids.

✦ Robin's Story

Robin was twenty-two years old when she consulted me because she was having no periods at all. She had begun to menstruate quite early, on her eleventh birthday. At first, her periods were very irregular and painful, so her mother took Robin to her own gynecologist. He prescribed birth control pills to regulate Robin's periods and reduce cramps. Robin stayed on the pill for several years, until she began experiencing disturbing negative symptoms. She felt as if her vision were deteriorating, and her contact lenses did not seem to fit anymore. She was also experiencing frequent headaches, and her moods became erratic just before her periods. Then her periods became nearly nonexistent. Robin also complained of a vague feeling that she was not quite herself anymore, especially on the days just before her period was expected. She decided to stop taking the pill. After several months without the pill, her periods still did not resume, so she came to see me.

During our history-taking session, Robin also complained of breast tenderness so severe that she sometimes could not even wear a bra, and the nagging and frequent sensation that her period was about to start. She also told me that she often woke up several times during the night, which left her exhausted during the day. The headaches that had forced her to give up the pill had changed in nature, but they had not disappeared, and she often craved carbohydrates. If she did give in and gorged on carbs, almost immediately after, she felt shaky and foggy-headed. Not surprisingly, Robin's relationship with her boyfriend was floundering because of her frequent temper flare-ups for no apparent reason. Robin was very athletic and had been on the girls' gymnastic team during college. Because of that sport's strict weight requirements, she still had very little body fat. I knew this was yet another contributing factor in a clear-cut case of severe hormonal imbalance.

Looking at Robin's history of irregular and painful menses as a young girl, plus several years on birth control pills, I suspected that she had not ovulated very much following her first few menstruations. She certainly had not menstruated normally at all during the years she was on the pill. Robin's symptoms all pointed to an estrogen-dominant state, a condition in which estrogen levels in the blood are not balanced out by sufficient progesterone. As I have already noted, an estrogen-dominant state can lead to several problems in later years, including gallbladder disturbances, blood sugar imbalances, osteoporosis, troublesome premenstrual syndrome, endometriosis, cervical dysplasia, infertility, and *fibroid tumors of the uterus*.

In order to keep herself from developing these disorders, Robin needed to take corrective steps. She eliminated all processed foods from her diet and increased her intake of essential fatty acids. I encouraged her to take supplements and herbs that would also help bring her body into better balance. Her program also included daily applications of natural progesterone cream for two to three weeks of each month, in order to supplement the hormone her body had lacked for so many years.

After several anxious months, Robin began feeling better. Soon, spontaneously, she began menstruating. That was a happy moment for both of us. I hoped that this early intervention would keep her on a healthy lifestyle to restore and maintain her hormonal balance and keep her healthy.

✦ Kelly's Story

As I noted in the beginning of this chapter, even stress can disrupt the delicate processes and balance maintained by the hormonal web. Take the case of Kelly, a forty-six-year-old attorney who was about to enter menopause. While she was happy not to be experiencing hot flashes, Kelly could not understand why her periods were getting heavier instead of scantier. Also, her abdomen was growing noticeably larger, even though she was not eating any more than usual. Before menopause, Kelly's periods arrived like clockwork, every twenty-eight days. Now, her periods were coming anywhere from eighteen to forty-eight days apart. Sometimes she could tell her period was coming because she experienced typical premenstrual symptoms. At other times, the bleeding would take her completely by surprise. The cramping and bleeding were becoming so severe that they interfered with her life. She was forced to carry tampons everywhere, and, on one occasion, the bleeding and cramping were so bad that she had to excuse herself from an important business meeting.

To make matters worse, Kelly was losing bladder control. She finally visited her gynecologist, who diagnosed her with one large subserous and several intramural fibroids. He recommended a hysterectomy.

Kelly's husband had died a few years earlier, leaving her with the responsibilities of being a busy attorney and a single mother to three school-age children. Live-in help was a necessity, but it was also a financial drain. In fact, when she finally took time to look back, Kelly realized that ever since her husband's passing and the increased pressures of her life, her periods had grown even more irregular and uncomfortable.

Although Kelly did not plan to bear more children, she did not want to lose her uterus and ovaries. She also wanted to improve her general health. A hysterectomy did not fit her plans. Nor could she possibly afford to take off any time from the demands of family and work to have surgery and recuperation. An associate, whom I had treated successfully for fibroids, suggested that Kelly consult me.

During our initial history-taking, I was struck by the fact that Kelly was on the threshold of menopause yet bleeding heavily during menstruation and not experiencing hot flashes. These symptoms pointed toward hormonal imbalance aggravated by the surge in estrogen levels that sometimes occurs just before menopause.

I also discovered that she had taken birth control pills for many years, and that her periods had been irregular only since her husband's death. Kelly followed what I call a typical standard American diet (SAD) that includes many fast foods. But equally important was the sharp increase of stress in Kelly's life and her inability to release that stress. When I mentioned this last point, Kelly seemed unaware that there are ways to nurture oneself and relieve stress.

Stress and Fibroids

Stress can be a subtle yet powerful factor in fibroid development and growth. This is because stress includes such psychological states as unresolved anger, fear, anxiety, worry, and other strong emotions governed by the so-called "primitive" limbic part of the brain. Remember: the limbic brain—the section of the brain located just above the hypothalamus—is also the first to set off the chain of hormonal cues that govern menstruation and other body processes. Chronic stress can impair the limbic brain's function, thereby disrupting the whole hormonal chain of command that continues with the pituitary, the hypothalamus, and the uterus and ovaries. Of course, these are the very same endocrine glands and organs that

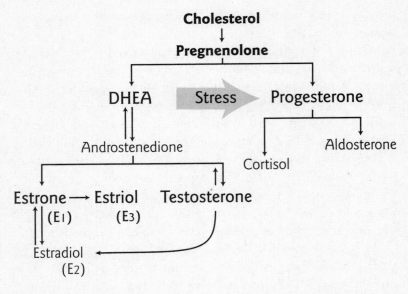

also govern your menstrual cycle and other body processes by maintaining proper hormone levels, releasing them with precise timing, and keeping each hormone in proper balance. This is how strong and persistent emotional disturbances can disrupt that hormonal balance. Once that balance is disturbed, fibroids can grow. In fact, hormonal imbalance could be the reason fibroids develop in the first place.

Constant and unrelieved stress also disturbs other hormone production, because stress has an adverse affect on the adrenal glands' production of the hormones cortisol, DHEA, and the so-called sex hormones.

Stress was clearly a major factor in Kelly's condition. Her fibroid uterus had swollen to the size of a thirteen-weeks pregnancy, but we were able to shrink it substantially by focusing on regulating her menstrual cycle through balancing her hormone levels. We did this with a comprehensive program that included the right nutrition, supplements, and herbs. Even more important was teaching Kelly how to manage and reduce the negative effects of stress. Gradually her symptoms subsided, and she was able to make a smooth transition into menopause. At that point, her estrogen and progesterone levels lowered, and her fibroids shrank even further.

The Limbic Brain System—Emotions and Fibroids

Let us take a closer look at how the limbic brain handles emotion. Following a route similar to the chain of hormonal commands that control menstruation and other body functions, the limbic system recognizes emotions and translates them via the hypothalamus to the pituitary gland. From there, the message of these emotions is passed on to the rest of the body. The body then responds to so-called negative emotions, such as fear and anger, with increased perspiration, heart and pulse rate, adrenal production, and decreased digestive rate—all symptoms of what is commonly called the basic "fight or flight" response. All these body responses are mediated by the chemical messengers we call neuropeptides and the hormones secreted by various endocrine glands. This is how strong emotion can interfere with balanced hormone production, by diverting energy from that job to the body responses that signal powerful emotion. Living in a chronic state of fear, worry, anxiety, or anger can create a state of hormonal imbalance that sets you up for fibroids.

Kelly was still mourning her husband, and she was also angry and fearful over the burden of supporting and raising three small children on her own. This powerful stew of emotions was clearly impairing her hormone production and balance. The signals from her limbic system to the hypothalamus and then, in turn, to the pituitary, and so on, were upsetting luteinizing hormone (LH) production to the point where she had stopped ovulating regularly. This created a state of estrogen dominance, in which overly high estrogen levels were not balanced out by appropriate levels of progesterone. The growth of the lining in the uterus that is stimulated by estrogen was not being turned off at the right time by the action of progesterone. This estrogen-progesterone imbalance meant that growth in other areas of the body was not turned off as well. This is how uterine smooth muscle cells can start growing in small, focused areas of the uterus. It is this kind of overgrowth that eventually becomes a fibroid.

Typically stressful events that set women up for fibroids and other conditions related to hormonal imbalance include the sudden onset of menopause that commonly follows the death of a spouse or parent. Women frequently experience irregular cycles when traveling, especially when they are in pressurized cabins on aircraft. Hormone irregularities often occur during college final exam week; periods of divorce, marriage, or job change; and difficult times with children.

The influence of the mind upon the body can be even more dramatic. This was brought home to me in the mid-eighties, when I agreed to give my first public talk on the holistic approach to women's health. I was terrified. I had absolutely no previous public speaking experience, and like most people, I feared making a fool of myself. Two weeks before my scheduled talk, I began to lose my voice toward the end of each day. The condition become increasingly severe, until I was forced to consult an ear, nose, and throat specialist. She was surprised to discover that I had grown a polyp on my vocal cords. She told me that she usually saw this condition in singers, people with a habit of screaming, and heavy smokers. I fit none of those categories, but my fear of public speaking was so great that my body had stepped in to the rescue. In order to remove the source of my fear—public speaking—it actually created a polyp on my vocal cord. The benign polyp had to be removed surgically, but its mission was accomplished: I was forced to cancel my talk. Needless to say, I eventually made the link between my fear and the polyp and worked on resolving the fear. I went on to deliver countless talks without ever losing my voice or growing another polyp.

The mind's control over the body is also illustrated in the well-known placebo effect. During double-blind, placebo-controlled studies for new drugs, patients do not know if they are receiving the real drug or an inactive substance known as the placebo. Yet 35 percent to 40 percent or more of the placebo group of patients consistently show improvement in their symptoms. This improvement is attributed to their *belief* that the substance they are taking will make them better. Surprisingly, conventional medicine does not assign this phenomenon much importance. It seems to me, though, that the placebo effect confirms the body's powerful ability to self-heal through the force of the mind's belief.

During the seventies, a drug called Laetrile, which was made from apricot pits, was widely touted as a miracle cancer cure. One patient experienced a fantastic response to Laetrile prescribed by a doctor who believed in the drug. After that same doctor was indoctrinated in conventional medical thinking, he reported to his patient that Laetrile was useless. The patient immediately experienced a total relapse.

Dr. Bernie Siegel relates many stories about patients who were given six months to live by their doctors and then obligingly died on the last day of the sixth month. In his practice—and in other practices founded on the mind-body interconnection and including healing visualizations and affirmations—these dire prognoses are often proved wrong.

Research conducted at the Institute of HeartMath in Boulder Creek, California, measured the effects of movie and TV violence, such as the violence depicted in a horror movie or on the six o'clock news, on the blood concentration of the hormone DHEA and the immunoglobulin secretory IgA. The study then contrasted those results with the effects on those same substances of images portraying love and caring, such as footage of Mother Teresa ministering to the poor and sick. DHEA is touted as the antiaging hormone and has been found to enhance immune system function, reduce incidence of cancer, and strengthen the adrenal glands. It is also a precursor to estrogen and testosterone, so it plays a key role in maintaining hormone levels and balance. Secretory IgA is the first of the body's protective immunoglobulins, or antibodies to interact with the outside world, because it is located on the mucous membranes that begin in the mouth and protect the entire intestinal tract. Low levels of secretory IgA leave an individual susceptible to infection from virtually every potentially infectious disease.

The institute published results indicating that the emotions set off in the viewer by images of violence reduce the levels of both DHEA and secretory IgA. When more pacific and loving emotions are stimulated in the viewer by viewing Mother Teresa, DHEA and secretory IgA levels rise!

Now, let us consider the fact that the age at which menses begins in American females has been lowering steadily over the past few decades. Today, the average age for onset of menses is twelve and one-half years. Fifty years ago, the average age was between fourteen and fifteen. Those of us working in the holistic medical field attribute at least part of this change to the increased exposure of young girls to media images of sex and violence. As you have just learned, exposure to violence has harmful effects on the immune system and on hormone balance.

If you want to explore the mind-body/body-mind connection further to learn how your mind affects your health, Barbara Levine's *Your Body Believes Every Word You Say* offers many examples of ways in which emotions control bodily function.

✦ Marianne's Story

Marianne had a twenty-two-weeks-size intramural and subserous fibroid uterus and was told in no uncertain terms that her only option was a hysterectomy. A forty-six-year-old businesswoman who managed a large, hectic office for a group of attorneys, Marianne had never married or had children, but she wanted to avoid surgery, even though, as her doctor commented, her uterus was an "unnecessary" organ for a woman of her age.

Marianne had no particular interest in holistic methods of healing. She did not even take a daily multivitamin. But I was her last chance to stay out of the operating room.

After examining Marianne and eliminating the possibility of a malignancy, we talked about her life and the possible role stress could be playing in exacerbating, perhaps even creating, severe imbalances in her hormone levels. A small cyst on her left ovary was additional evidence of hormone imbalance.

Marianne started out with a simplified version of the healing program, which included dietary changes, vitamins, herbs, and learning how to meditate with tapes that I recommended. When Marianne returned to see me eight weeks later, her fibroid uterus had shrunk dramatically, to eighteen-weeks size, and Marianne told me that she was feeling "wonderful." Eight weeks later, her fibroid uterus had shrunk down to sixteen-weeks size. While we were discussing how happy we both were with this result, Marianne suddenly burst out, "I've had it with this job! I'm not being appreciated! I'm being taken for granted! It has been so stressful, and I'm suddenly realizing that it's time for me to move on." The healing program had focused on healing Marianne's physical health, but the tremendous amount of stress attached to her job was another major factor in her fibroid condition. Once Marianne confronted this fact, she realized that she could eliminate a great deal of stress—along with its toxic effects on her body—by leaving her job.

Now that you have a picture of how the vast and intricate hormonal web interconnects your body and mind, you can better appreciate why the most effective way to address your fibroid condition is through a holistic treatment plan that will restore you to total health.

PART TWO

THE HOLISTIC VIEW

3

Optimum Health

You have learned about the connection between fibroids and conditions of hormonal imbalance that adversely affect your health in many possible ways. You have heard about an ideal condition described here as optimal health. By now, you may be wondering about this optimum health. What exactly is it?

From the holistic point of view, optimum health is a state of aliveness, wholeness, and balance that promotes peak function of body, mind, and spirit. From this broad and inclusive point of view, a single health issue such as uterine fibroids cannot truly be healed, as long as the function of your body, mind, or spirit is still compromised in any way.

If the condition is not treated holistically, either fibroids will recur or the disharmony will express itself as another health disorder.

Optimum health rests on a three-cornered foundation:
1. Unconditional love of your body, mind, and spirit
2. Awareness of self and others
3. Acceptance of responsibility for your own health

Holistic medicine reflects that foundation in its four core principles:
1. Promote unconditional love for one's self and others, which is life's most powerful healer

2. Address the whole person—body, mind, and spirit
3. Integrate conventional and complementary medical therapies
4. Employ treatments that balance attention to relieving symptoms with the ultimate objective of discovering and healing
   root problems of the disorder

Women come to me for help with problems that they consider to be purely gynecological, among them, vaginitis, vaginal discharge, abnormal bleeding, endometriosis, cervical dysplasia, PMS, symptoms of menopause, lower abdominal pain that they attribute to reproductive organs, chronic bladder infections, and, of course, fibroid tumors. Whatever their problem, they usually believe it is solely related to their gynecological function. Yet, after I take their history, I invariably discover that their pelvic organs are not the real causes of their problems. The true reason for any of these bodily complaints is that some aspect of their lives is out of balance.

✦ Delores's Story

Delores was a woman in her late thirties, married to a man who often traveled for work, leaving her alone at home with three children all under the age of ten. Apparently, there was no extra money for outside housekeeping or baby-sitting help. Of course, Delores did not come to me to consult on her family life. She was in my office because her periods had been getting increasingly irregular. By the time of her first visit, they were coming anywhere from eighteen to thirty-five days apart, and Delores was often taken by surprise by the onset of bleeding. Previously, her periods had been extremely regular. Now, the bleeding was quite scanty at times, while at others, the flow was so profuse that tampons and sanitary pads were not enough. She told me that recently she had been forced to stand in the shower and let the blood drip down her legs and wash away. The bleeding was often so profuse that Delores felt utterly drained. She feared blacking out, with no one there to help.

Delores was also experiencing painful periods for the first time. She had to take Advil every four hours just to get through some days. Worst of all, she found that she could no longer tolerate her children. She often found herself screaming and yelling over the most minor infractions, especially during those three or four days when she knew her period was about to arrive. Still, Delores's major concern was the excessive and irregular bleeding. Her mother had died of some female-system-related cancer—she did not know exactly what—and Delores was terrified that she was destined for the same fate. In fact, immediately after describing her health complaints, Delores wanted to know if she would have to have a dilation and curettage (D&C)—also known as a scraping of the uterus—or some other surgery.

Delores conformed to the general image most of us have of the typical homemaker, the kind of woman who has learned from her mother that her role is nurturer of the family. Most of the time, Delores nurtured her children very well, and she also took care of her husband when he was home. In fact, everyone but Delores was very well cared for. Delores never seemed to find time to do anything for herself. When I asked what she did for her own pleasure, she gave me a blank look. Then, as a tear came to her eye, she answered, "Nothing."

What do *you* do for your own enjoyment? If you are like Delores, always taking care of others, never finding time for yourself, let her example be your wake-up call. One of the strongest indicators of massive imbalance within your system is an inability to find enjoyment in your day-to-day life.

So-called free time was not spent putting up her feet, exercising, or reading a book. "Free time" in Delores's dictionary meant a chance to catch up on laundry, keep the home in order, and drive the children from one activity to the next. When Delores told me that her normal bowel movements occurred once or twice a week, I was not surprised. She did not even give herself enough time for a daily bowel movement!

Many years of this elimination pattern had left Delores with a severe constipation problem. Yet she viewed her lifestyle as normal. We have already seen how an abnormal intestinal environment, or intestinal dysbiosis, can impact hormone balance.

Delores's eating habits showed a similar lack of self-care. Whenever her husband was on the road, which was most of the time, Delores ate at the kitchen counter while preparing meals for the children. She would just throw whatever she was making for the kids into her mouth and rarely sat down for a quiet meal. That meant that Delores's diet consisted of the typical meals consumed by Americans under ten years old: chicken fingers, hot dogs, French fries, and pasta, all liberally dosed with ketchup. At least the French fries and ketchup gave her two of the suggested minimum of five vegetables and fruits per day.

Bob, Delores's husband, was busy traveling his sales territory for a men's clothing line, and Delores had no other family nearby to give her a hand. Since Bob supported the family financially, he did not believe Delores needed any help with her own work: taking care of him, the house, and the children. After all, his mother took care of his father and their family, so why shouldn't his own wife do the same? When Bob said there was not enough money for extra help, she believed him. She felt guilty for even suggesting in the first place that she might have help. In general, Delores viewed any request for herself as selfish.

When Bob was home, after he had eaten the dinner Delores served him, he would watch a sports event on TV while Delores washed dishes or performed another domestic chore. Periodically, he would ask her to "dial a number for me" or "make me a snack," and Delores always complied.

Delores had learned at a very early age that she was responsible for everyone else's needs. She'd grown up as the oldest child of three in a blue-collar family. Her father was an alcoholic, her mother was chronically ill, and Delores was seven years older than the second child. As far back as she could remember, she was diapering and feeding babies, as well as seeing to her parents' needs. When Delores left her family to marry, she chose a husband who was very similar to her demanding father.

After I finished taking Delores's history and learning about her present life, I performed a physical exam. My immediate concern, given Delores's abnormal bleeding, irregularity, and pain, was that her fibroid condition might be of the aborting submucous type. If that was true, surgery would be her sole option. The exam showed that her uterus was enlarged to the size of an eight- to ten-weeks pregnancy. An ultrasound exam showed the presence of intramural and subserous fibroids but no submucous fibroids. But it also revealed a questionable irregularity within the uterus, so I performed a sonohysterogram. This is an office sonogram performed while instilling normal saline (a sterile saltwater solution) into the uterus, in order to visualize the endometrium, or uterine lining. A simple office biopsy of the endometrium ruled out the possibility that the irregularity in the uterine lining could be a cancerous or precancerous condition called hyperplasia. Hyperplasia is an ongoing condition of excessive tissue growth within the uterus that can be simple—that is, benign—or atypical, which means that it is potentially precancerous.

After Delores got dressed, she came back into the consultation room to discuss what might be going on.

"Delores, we're going to wait until the biopsy report comes back for a definite answer on whether or not there's a premalignancy or malignancy," I said. "I'm fairly certain this is not the case and that your real problem is a hormone imbalance."

Delores looked very relieved. "Are you sure?" she asked.

"I'm not one hundred percent certain," I told her, "but given your age, what I could see on the sonogram, and the current statistics, everything suggests that this isn't going to be a malignancy. Besides, the rest of your history—your diet, your lifestyle, your constant state of physical and emotional stress, and the lack of emotional support—makes you a textbook case for hormonal imbalance.

"I'm not just talking about your female hormones," I explained. "I suspect that you also are suffering from weakness in your adrenal glands. These are the glands that help you deal with stress during moment-to-moment situations. Women who are under constant stress often exhaust their adrenals, and then the adrenal glands are not even able to deal with life's usual pressures and stressors, let alone produce certain hormones.

"This is one of the reasons why you're so anxious and irritable," I went on. "Adrenal weakness can also lead to poor sleep and fatigue during the day. We will also evaluate your thyroid gland, because there's a close relationship between all the endocrine glands and the various hormones they secrete. Whenever one gland is functioning out of balance, the other glands are often out of whack as well. We're going to take blood for a panel of tests to check for thyroid gland dysfunction before you leave today. After I get the results, we'll talk again. In the meantime, there are certain steps you can take right away that will help matters quite a bit."

At this point, Delores and I discussed what she could do to bring more balance into her life. Although I had many areas of concern in terms of her lifestyle, I felt that one of the most important changes she could make would be to find a little time to nurture herself, to do anything just for her own enjoyment. She was not going to leave my office and head straight for a yoga class, but I recommended a meditation tape series that is very easy to follow. All she would have to do was sit down alone for five to ten minutes a day and listen to this soothing tape. I also showed her a ten-to-fifteen-minute yoga stretch routine. We discussed the importance of improving her diet and eating habits, as well as the importance of regular, daily bowel movements. Again, the key here was making time for herself. Finally, I recommended a few nutrients and herbs to support her system. (You will learn in detail about these foods, supplements, and herbs in Chapters 4, 5, and 6.)

When the biopsy came back, it showed no trace of cancer or a precancerous condition. It did indicate hormonal imbalance, though, because there was no evidence of progesterone effect. (As you know from Chapter 2, no evidence of progesterone's effect on the body meant that Delores was not ovulating.) In other words, she was in an estrogen-dominant condition, one that made her ripe for the development of fibroids and additional gynecological disorders as she grew older. The blood tests confirmed many of my other suspicions.

Her thyroid was not functioning well. I use the thyroid stimulating hormone (TSH) test, which indicates how hard the pituitary gland has to work in order to stimulate the thyroid to produce thyroid hormones. If there is not a lot of thyroid hormone being produced, the TSH level will be high, which means the pituitary is working harder than normal to get the thyroid going. More significantly, a high TSH level means that the thyroid gland is not producing enough hormones, a condition known as hypothyroidism, or low thyroid. This is an example of the intricate and precise weave of the hormonal web, especially the feedback loop that governs the menstrual cycle. In the case of this particular phase of the feedback loop, the pituitary gland stimulates the thyroid gland to make more hormones whenever body levels are low. If thyroid hormones are high, the pituitary gland lowers that stimulation to normal levels. So, low TSH levels indicate an overactive thyroid state, which is called hyperthyroidism, or Graves' disease. Contrary to popular belief, you do not have to have a goiter or swelling on the neck from thyroid enlargement to be suffering from thyroid dysfunction.

Although Delores's TSH level was in the normal range, it fell into what I consider the high normal range. This condition often sets in when the inactive form of thyroid hormone known as thyroxin (T4) is in the normal range, but there is not adequate conversion of that inactive thyroid hormone into the active thyroid hormone known as triiodothyronine (T3). For this reason, I also routinely check blood levels of free or total T3, to learn if adequate conversion of inactive to active thyroid hormone is taking place. Many possible nutritional and hormonal deficiencies can interfere with this conversion.

Whenever I perform a physical examination, I look for the physical signs that suggest a sluggish thyroid. Three of those signs relate to the thyroid hormone's ability to convert the beta-carotene in fruits and vegetables into the form of vitamin A the body can use. One sign of a low or malfunctioning thyroid hormone is the presence of those small bumps on the back of the arm that feel like goose bumps, or "chicken skin." Medicine calls the condition hypertrophic folliculitis, or vitamin A bumps. A second sign that a woman may not have sufficiently active thyroid hormone is yellow-tinged palms, because the precursor to vitamin A is being deposited in that area of the body instead of changing into A and being used. The third dependable sign of possible low thyroid hormone function is a noticeable slowing of the Achilles tendon reflex.

I noticed that Delores had vitamin A bumps on the backs of her arms and a slowing of her Achilles tendon reflex. As I suspected, the blood tests confirmed that Delores had low levels of active T3. I wanted to evaluate her thyroid function more specifically, so I asked her to do a basal body temperature test every morning, for five days in a row at the beginning of her menstrual cycle. This effective means of evaluating thyroid function was originally proposed by Dr. Broda Barnes in his book *Hypothyroidism: The Unsuspected Illness*. The patient takes her underarm temperature first thing every morning for seven minutes. If the average temperature over five days is less than 97.4, a hypothyroid state, or underactive thyroid, is suspected. This is based on the correlation between thyroid function, basal metabolic rate, and basal temperature. Women who are menstruating take their temperature every morning during the first five days of their cycle. If they take their temperatures later on in their cycle, the normal rise in temperature that occurs with ovulation due to the effect of progesterone will not give an accurate result. (Incidentally, that rise in temperature indicates that an egg has been released from an ovary.) Postmenopausal women can take their temperatures at any time during the month for a period of five days.

Delores was so unaccustomed to taking time for herself that she actually struggled to perform this test. Lying in bed for seven minutes was a challenge in itself, so I encouraged her to take that time to play the meditation tapes I'd recommended. The test also became added incentive for Delores to lie still and quiet her mind for several minutes. As I had suspected, her basal temperature averaged 96.7, suggesting a mild condition of hypothyroidism.

The healing program I devised for Delores took into account not only the results of these fairly conventional medical tests, as well as the information I had gathered about her life. I was completely certain on one point, that a D&C or any other invasive surgical measure, including a hysterectomy, would do nothing to remedy Delores's real and underlying problem, the pervasive theme of imbalance that ran throughout Delores's life.

Let us return for a moment to the four principles of holistic medicine:

1. Promote unconditional love for one's own body
2. Address the needs of body, mind, and spirit
3. Integrate conventional and complementary therapies
4. Balance attention to relief of symptoms with treatment of root causes

Delores and I worked together, following these holistic health principles, to create a healing program that would maximize her health, resolve her problem of excessive bleeding, and correct the estrogen-dominant state associated with her fibroid condition.

At first, the notion of self-nurturing or self-love was completely foreign to her. "It feels like being selfish," she commented to me. I decided to tell her about another patient whom I had once tried to help with the same issue.

Ruth was a sixty-five-year-old woman who had undergone a successful operation for ovarian cancer. Several years later, though, she began complaining of abdominal pain and swelling in her belly. Tests revealed that the cancer had recurred, and Ruth was put on an intensive program of chemotherapy. At first, Ruth responded well to the chemo, but then she suffered a massive relapse, with large accumulations of fluid in her abdomen, a condition called acites.

I met Ruth at this low point, when I consulted on her case in the hospital. I was immediately struck by how sad, depressed, and lonely Ruth seemed, and I began visiting her almost every afternoon, just to talk and keep her company. Something about Ruth provoked my empathy, and I genuinely cared about her. Over the course of our chats, I learned that Ruth had been the homemaker and nurturer of her family and was always too busy caring for others to nurture herself. Ultimately, she revealed to me that she did not even know how to accept nurturing or love from anyone, and her family's gestures of concern and care made her acutely uncomfortable. Ruth believed it was her duty to give her husband and children all her love and attention and receive nothing in return. I tried to explain that now she needed to accept their love and nurturing in order to heal. I met with her family and was impressed by their genuine love for her. They all desired to give back to Ruth some of the care she had given them. We spent many days discussing this issue, but Ruth steadfastly refused even to try accepting their love and nurturing. Whenever they came with gifts, she would reject them, saying she did not need them. More important, whenever they wanted to spend time with her and lend their help, she would send them home with protestations that she was fine and wanted to be alone to rest. "Anyway," she would always say, "you need to take care of yourself!"

Ruth finally realized that if she did not accept her family's love and nurturing, she would not survive. Yet, she was still too uncomfortable with accepting their care to let them in. Sadly, Ruth died without ever allowing her family to express their love and caring.

Of course, Ruth may have died of the cancer anyway. But studies suggest that embracing her family's nurturing and love would have given Ruth, at very the least, a little more time at a much better quality of life. Several breast cancer studies show that women who participate in support groups enjoy longer cancer-free periods and live higher-quality lives than women who do not experience that support. In the mid-seventies, a psychiatrist at Stanford University named David Spiegel conducted a compelling study on women whose breast cancers had spread throughout their bodies. He randomly assigned some women to discussion groups, while others did not participate in any groups. Spiegel hoped to prove that the opportunity to share and discuss daily issues reduces the emotional distress of coping with breast cancer. His intention was not to prove that the interaction between mind and body affects physical health. In fact, Spiegel's first publications of his study results suggested nothing more than that the women reported feeling "better" because they could "vent" their emotions in supportive settings. The real surprise arrived ten years later, after the experiment concluded and his data was completely analyzed. Spiegel discovered that the women who participated in the support groups lived an average of eighteen months longer and reported a better quality of life than those women not assigned to groups.

Other studies show that men who are single or divorced suffer higher accident and suicide rates and more heart disease than men who are in successful relationships. At the University of California, San Francisco, epidemiologist Maradee Davis studied over 7,500 adult men between the ages of forty-five and fifty-four. She discovered that those who were single had a two times greater chance of dying within the next ten years than married men of the same age. Other studies even indicate that people who have relationships with pets enjoy healthier, longer, happier lives. In one such study, 345 elderly pet owners were found to visit their doctors less often than a comparable group who did not own pets.

All this data convinces me that even if Ruth had not been cured of her cancer, those last months in the hospital might have been months or years spent at home, enjoying the warm embrace of her loving family.

After I finished recounting Ruth's sad tale, Delores closed her eyes and thought for a moment. "I think I see what you mean," she finally said. "If I were that sick, I would have a hard time letting other people take care of me, too. But I understand your point: if I don't start taking care of myself now and asking for some help without feeling as if I'm selfish, who knows what could happen to me! I definitely want to be healthier, and I sure don't want to get sicker."

I explained that taking care of herself was not selfish at all. In fact, it would be a positive act of love for her children and her husband, although, admittedly, Bob would probably be hard to convince. I told Delores that people who are capable of nurturing themselves and others and are able to express love through compassionate action also experience higher self-esteem and happiness. I explained how children learn from their parents' example. Seeing their mother taking care of herself would give Delores's children a model of how they could care for themselves as healthy, well-balanced adults. Awakening their sense of responsibility by assigning them chores around the house would give them a healthy dose of independence and accomplishment and teach them the value of being accountable for their actions. Delores finally realized that she could unload at least part of her burden without being selfish, as long as she did so with love. It would be a win-win situation for all concerned.

As predicted, Bob was a bit harder to convince. In fact, the transition to this healthier phase in their relationship had to be smoothed with the help of a marriage counselor. After several months of witnessing the positive effects of his changed family structure on his happier, healthier wife and his less demanding and whiny children, Bob eventually came around.

Learning how to love and nurture herself and accept help from her family helped fulfill the second and third principles of Delores's holistic healing: addressing the needs of the whole person, including mind and spirit.

The needs of her body had brought her in to see me, but Delores soon realized that true healing meant taking care of the needs of her mind and spirit as well. Her body's needs were addressed by changes in her diet, detoxification programs, intestinal support, the use of supplements and herbs, adequate rest, and regular exercise. She also learned about environmental toxins and became mindful of ways to eliminate them from her life. (In Chapter 2, I described briefly how environmental toxins that behave in your body like false hormones can be a major contributor to medical conditions related to hormonal imbalance and toxic overload. Chapter 8 describes these toxins in greater detail and tells you how you can lessen their harmful effects and cut down their presence in your personal environment.)

The meditation tapes and yoga stretches I recommended to Delores were a great first step toward correcting and preventing the ravages of daily stress. After Delores got used to taking time out for destressing techniques, I introduced her to the even more powerful healing benefits of positive visualizations and statements of healing affirmation. Together, we developed a visualization script that addressed her specific needs and objectives and was filled with affirmations for her healing. She recorded the script onto a tape cassette that she played every day to herself as she relaxed. I told her that the script and tape were her own production. They could be edited and rewritten to suit any problems, on any level. At the same time that Delores relaxed and played her positive visualization tape every day, she also applied castor oil packs to her lower abdomen. This effective healing remedy, developed by the famous "Sleeping Prophet," Edgar Cayce, advances the healing of many different abdominal disorders. I have discovered that combining the castor oil packs—which you will learn how to use in Chapter 9—with positive visualizations and affirmations, makes for a powerful healing tool. These meditation/castor-oil-pack sessions addressed Delores's physical, emotional, and spiritual needs, because affirmations and visualizations are believed to draw on universal healing energy. Not only does that energy enter into your individual being, it promotes your sense of being an integral part of a unified, harmonious existence.

In keeping with the third principle of holistic healing, Delores's program drew on both conventional and holistic medical knowledge. My evaluation of Delores's health problems was based on proven conventional medical tests. At the same time, I used all my conventional and holistic training and years of clinical experience to identify the root causes of her individual condition. Few conventional gynecologists venture outside the female organs to look for possible contributing factors rooted in diet patterns, gastrointestinal function, lifestyle, family situations, and other areas that make up virtually every aspect of a patient's life. Yet many of these seemingly unrelated considerations can have a direct and profound influence on gynecological disorders like fibroid tumors.

Because conventional medicine has such a narrow focus, it offered Delores little in the way of "cures," other than drugs and various surgical procedures. Although drugs can relieve some symptoms, they do nothing to address and correct the root causes of the condition. The drugs can also create negative effects, all of which may not yet be known. Ironically, these effects often dictate the use of even more drugs. By the time a typical chronically ill patient reaches her sixties, she has been introduced to the concept of polypharmacy. She is on a daily regimen of many drugs, some of which are actually prescribed to offset the negative effects of the others.

Delores's therapy was holistic in every sense of the term, because it drew from conventional and natural or complementary therapies, not only to relieve symptoms but also to address causes on every possible level. Once her fibroids were under control, the problem would not rear its head again.

Delores worked on herself in partnership with me, and, after one year, she was well on her way to achieving that primary objective of holistic medicine: optimal health of body, mind, and spirit. The problem that had brought Delores to my office—irregular, painful periods—had been resolved. Delores was back to regular cycles, no longer hemorrhaging, and rarely experiencing cramps. Even the nagging skin conditions that she never even thought to mention—after all, I'm not a dermatologist!—cleared up, thanks to her improved diet and nutrient program. Her moods were now consistently appropriate, and she enjoyed her life and her family much more. She was taking care of herself with regular yoga classes. She had also joined a women's book club and was enjoying pleasurable, supportive relationships with her new friends. Delores reported that she felt more positive and calm in general, in part, because she was keeping up her meditation and visualization practice. Bob was also healthier and happier, because their life together had grown much more fulfilling.

4

The Fibroid-Healing Diet

Let food be your medicine, and let medicine be your food.
—HIPPOCRATES, *father of modern medicine*

Flaxseed and soybean products instead of hormone therapy or birth control pills to regulate and balance your hormone levels? A dairy-free diet to restore gynecological health? That's right! Eating smart is one of your most powerful weapons in your fight against fibroid tumors.

By now, you understand how the holistic view of health—including body, mind, and spirit—connects to healthy hormone function. In this chapter, you will learn how hormone function is closely linked to the types of foods you eat, their quality, and the ways in which they are prepared, digested, and assimilated into your body.

You are what you eat. You have heard that old axiom before, but the subject of nutrition is so important to your health that I had to state it again. On one hand, nutritious food is your best health protector and restorer. Crucial nutrients in food protect and boost your overall health and vitality, at the same time that they prevent and heal gynecological conditions, including the development of fibroids.

The Standard American Diet: SAD

An unhealthy diet robs your body of the nutrients it needs to function at peak strength, maintain hormone balance, and prevent related diseases. Inadequate nutrition weakens your entire body—brain, nerves, genitals, endocrine glands, heart, blood vessels, liver, gastrointestinal tract, and everything else, leaving you vulnerable to widespread imbalance and disease.

Jonathan Wright, M.D., one of the leading nutritionally oriented physicians in this country, describes those who eat what has become standard fare in America as "the Pepsi degeneration." Others, including myself, describe the Standard American Diet as SAD.

Too many of us fuel our rushed, pressure-filled modern lives with fast foods: soft drinks made of little more than sugar or artificial sweeteners, bottomless cups of coffee, unhealthy saturated fats, empty carbohydrates, and harmful chemical additives. These "foods" may give us a quick burst of energy, but they offer very little real nutrition beyond that initial jolt. In the end, those who stick to the SAD are like someone who keeps withdrawing money from the bank without making sufficient deposits to ensure funds will always be there.

If you are on the SAD—eating the wrong foods instead of foods that build health—you are eroding your overall physical resources, vitality, disease resistance, and your gynecological health. If you are young, you probably have not felt the harmful effects of your substandard diet. Wait ten, twenty, or thirty years, when that inadequate nutritional investment will leave you shortchanged. Your only dividends will be deteriorated health, chronic fatigue, frequent infections, and a host of medical conditions related to poor immunity, weakened endocrine glands, and hormonal imbalance, including fibroids.

A Nation of Tired People

Health-care providers report that the number one health complaint today is lack of energy. Many of the patients who come to my office because of gynecological disorders such as fibroids also complain of poor hair quality, dry and flaking skin, digestive difficulties of all kinds, sleep disorders, frequent infections and colds, and low vitality. They believe that all they need is a prescription for a new miracle drug. Some actually become angry when I suggest that what they really need is a change of diet. When they finally do make necessary adjustments in their eating habits, they are often astounded by how much better they feel. After only four weeks of healthier eating, their hair, skin, and nails become healthy and glowing. Sleep patterns and energy levels improve, and lifelong digestive problems disappear. Eventually, fibroids stop growing and sometimes even shrink.

The real miracle drug isn't a drug; it's good food. All it takes is eating health-giving foods, and you are on your way to greater vitality and healing. Follow the nutritional advice you are about to discover, and you will be taking an important step toward greater health and restoring your hormones to the state of balance that prevents and heals fibroid conditions.

It's all up to you.

✦ Louise's Story

Louise, a thirty-year-old overweight African-American woman, visited her regular gynecologist for a routine checkup. Much to her surprise, he reported that several intramural fibroids had expanded her uterus to the size of a ten-weeks pregnancy. Louise's periods were normal and she was symptom-free, but she was concerned about the possible effects on future childbearing. She was plagued with terrifying childhood memories of her mother's emergency hysterectomy. Louise never did find out why her mother had the surgery, but she would never forget her mother's terrible pain and all that bleeding. Louise did not want to inherit her mother's fate.

On taking Louise's history, I discovered that her fibroids could be thriving thanks to her SAD program. Louise lived on fast food—hamburgers, French fries, sodas, and milk shakes. Let us take a look at the other foods consumed on a typically SAD day:

SAD BREAKFAST

Doughnuts and coffee are a favorite SAD breakfast. Variations on that theme can include a bagel with cream cheese, butter, or margarine (under the mistaken belief that margarine protects your heart). You might have cereal made from sugared refined carbohydrates with milk containing traces of hormone, pesticide, and insecticides, or a hearty meal of fried bacon and eggs. Even worse, breakfast could be just a couple of cups of coffee to flog your already exhausted adrenal glands into action for the day. None of these choices offer any real nutritional value. In fact, all these foods are full of sugar, refined carbs, "bad" fats, and/or chemical additives that have been implicated in the chronic states of hormonal imbalance that promote fibroid growth.

Let's talk about coffee. Advertisements portray coffee as a warm, inclusive ritual of companionship: the husband and wife sharing a morning cup of coffee in a sunlit kitchen, friends gathering during the afternoon or evening over designer cappuccinos in a chic coffee bar. The truth about coffee is not as pleasant.

Coffee's kick comes from a very powerful drug to which many women are unknowingly addicted. Yes, the caffeine in a cup of coffee stimulates a burst of energy and boosts mental acuity. But that "lift" comes at a steep price. Coffee stimulates more than the adrenal glands to give you that energy rush. It also acts on the brain, the heart (causing cardiac rhythm irregularities), muscles, and kidneys (increasing the frequency of urination, which interrupts nighttime sleep). I can personally attest to the fact that a single cup of coffee is enough to cause a long sleepless night—and that's not all.

Caffeine has been implicated in breast fibrocystic problems, and it can influence the production and balance of hormones through its adverse effect on the body's ability to create and use the prostaglandins that it uses to make hormones. Caffeine also promotes hormonal imbalance by compromising the liver's ability to metabolize estrogens. It can interfere with the body's absorption of iron—a major problem for women who suffer from fibroid-induced anemia due to heavy bleeding.

Some women tell me that they drink only decaffeinated coffee, but even decaf can cause problems for a susceptible woman. If you do not know whether you are addicted to caffeine, try giving it up for a few days. If you do not get a headache within three days, caffeine is probably not harmful to you. If you are afflicted by one of those raging caffeine-withdrawal headaches, you are addicted to this drug, and it would be in your best interest to wean yourself off it. During the withdrawal period, be sure to drink plenty of water, at least half an ounce for every pound of your body weight. You can also try "nervine" type herbal teas like oat straw, chamomile, vervain, or valerian. For some of you, simply eliminating caffeine from your diet will be a major step toward better gynecological health.

SAD LUNCH

The most popular SAD lunches are probably a couple slices of pizza and a soda (more caffeine!), often consumed at the desk while working, or a quick bite under "Mickey D's Golden Arches." How about a double bacon cheeseburger, French fries cooked in animal fat, and a diet coke (to cut down on calories and fill you up with toxic chemicals)? The aspartame in the diet soft drink is another health threat. Studies show that aspartame, commonly known by the NutraSweet brand name, can instigate many health problems. "I get lunch from the salad bar," you may be protesting. That salad bar may seem like a healthful alternative, but if you load up on the wrong foods, it is just one baby step above a Double Whopper or a slice. Those wrong choices typically include heavily sugared low-fat dressings, bacon bits, and prepared salads loaded with mayonnaise. Most salad bars also offer heavy doses of additives, preservatives, and artificial colorings and flavorings that are supposed to boost gustatory appeal. No one can state with 100 percent certainty that these artificial chemicals promote hormone imbalance and fibroid growth, but they are among the leading suspects. Here is my rule of thumb: If it ain't natural to the human body, stay away from it.

SAD DINNER

Most people try to make better food choices for dinner. Unfortunately, dinner is often the largest meal of the day, even though evening activity for most Americans is nothing more taxing than clicking the remote in front of the TV and walking back and forth from the living room to the kitchen and bathroom. For most people on the SAD program, dinner is usually poultry or red meat, a vegetable, and a starch. That does not sound too bad, but the poultry and beef are commercially raised, which means they are chock-full of hormones, antibiotics, and pesticide residues. These chemicals are added to commercially prepared animal feed in order to make the animals fatter and to prevent disease. The more meat per animal, the greater the profit. Risk of infection is especially high for commercially raised animals and poultry because they are kept virtually immobile, crammed together in small cages and pens to save space. In addition, fast-food chicken and other meats are often smothered with a heavy, sugared barbecue sauce or dredged in flour and then fried in unhealthful saturated oils. Vegetables are a great idea, but if they are canned, frozen, or overcooked, they contain fewer nutrients. If they are commercially grown, they contain pesticide and insecticide residues. The meal's starch—let's say, rice—is usually refined, a process that leaches it of any nutritional value.

What is going on in American kitchens? Moms these days work nine-to-five jobs just like Dads, so there just isn't enough time to prepare a home-cooked meal from scratch. This is one reason why so many families depend on the fast-food industry for their "home cooking." Single career women and single mothers also slip into that "easy fixin' " routine, because their time is equally limited.

SAD SNACKS

While one hand operates the TV remote, the other hand is often busy dipping into bags of chips and/or pretzels. These "foods" consist mainly of unhealthful starch, oil, and salt. Chips, pretzels, and many other SAD snacks are so loaded with sodium that they make you thirsty, and that thirst is usually quenched with the SAD beverage of choice, the "soft" drinks consumed by "the Pepsi degeneration." Those drinks are also full of sodium, so if you drink one, you are soon ready to down another. Each can or bottle of soda also gives you several teaspoons of sugar or the equivalent of the dangerous sugar substitute aspartame. Even bottled and canned juice drinks, which some people mistakenly consider healthful, contain very little fruit, no fiber at all, and much too much sugar. Not enough Americans quench their thirst with the most healthful beverage of all, pure water. Other popular SAD snacks include pastries and ice cream or frozen yogurt—all are packed with saturated fats; sugar and/or refined starch; and the same antibiotic, pesticide, and hormone residues found in all commercially prepared dairy products.

Experts estimate that each American consumes an average of 140 pounds of sugar a year! I consume almost no sugar at all, having lost my taste for very sweet things after many years of cultivating healthful eating habits. I guess this means that one of you out there is gobbling up my allotment, giving you a whopping annual sugar intake of 280 pounds.

YOU'VE BEEN HAD

Amazingly, the refined and processed foods that constitute the bulk of the SAD program are stripped of essential nutrients and then enriched with chemical equivalents of those same nutrients that were taken out! In *Sugar Blues,* a seminal book on nutrition, author William Dufty writes, "If Dracula came in and sucked your blood and then gave you a B_{12} shot, would you say you'd been enriched or you'd been had?"

Let us take a closer look at this issue to discover exactly how you've been had and what's been stolen from your food.

The *B vitamins* that are removed during the processing of grains are essential for energy production in the body. If you are trying to stop fibroid growth, you need B vitamins like B_6 so your liver can metabolize estrogen efficiently and help restore hormone balance. Artificial colorings like *tartrazine,* which is commonly added to processed foods, act as vitamin B_6 antagonists, which means that tartrazine, *hydrazine,* and other artificial colorings, flavorings, and preservatives have profoundly negative effects on your body's ability to process and use vitamin B_6. These artificial food chemicals actually impair hormone metabolism. Some food additives are even more dangerous. Animal studies suggest that artificial colorings, such as red dye #3 and others used widely to make foods more attractive, are potentially carcinogenic. This means that they cause cells, both normal and cancerous ones, to grow. They can actually increase the size of tumors, including fibroids. They should be strictly avoided. Preservatives are supposed to promote long shelf life for processed foods and keep bugs away. If the bugs will not eat it because it has been there for months and months, why should you or I?

Essential minerals like *magnesium* and *zinc* are also removed during food processing. Those two minerals alone are responsible for at least five hundred different and essential reactions within your body. This is because magnesium and zinc act as chemical catalysts, increasing the efficiency and effectiveness of essential body reactions. Yet it has been estimated that as many as 70 percent of people who subsist on the SAD are deficient in magnesium and zinc. These people do not even consume the government recommended daily allowance (RDA) for magnesium and zinc.

My suggestion for strategic supermarket shopping is to stay only on the aisles at the periphery of the supermarket. That is where they keep fresh fruits and produce. Avoid the middle aisles, where most foods are bagged, boxed, or canned. If it does not grow naturally in nature, I do not eat it. Have you ever seen a potato chip tree? Actually, I recommend that you do not shop in standard supermarkets at all, because they offer very little food containing the quality nutrients you need to maintain or restore health and to heal fibroids. One welcome sign, though, is that more and more standard supermarkets are stocking their shelves with natural and organic products. Also, more nationwide chains of a new breed of natural foods supermarkets, like Fresh Fields and Bread and Circus, are catering to those demanding wholesome, unprocessed foods. With just a little effort on your part, you can find a natural foods market in your area. You can even order food from mail order catalogs and the Internet. (See the appendix.)

If you are saving time with the quick 'n' easy SAD program, you are putting yourself and your family at risk for serious health problems. The SAD way of eating gives you plenty of what you do not need and very little of what you do need: fiber, vitamins, minerals, health-promoting essential fats, complex carbohydrates, and lean protein that is free of antibiotic, pesticide, and hormone residues.

Remember Louise, the woman who was surprised to discover that she had a fibroid condition? The first time Louise consulted me about her fibroids, she was still symptom-free, but her SAD plan had already resulted in subtle negative effects on her health. The signs of those effects told me that it was only a matter of time before her fibroids became a serious problem. I discussed the fibroid-healing diet with Louise, but she was horrified by the prospect of making such a drastic alteration in her lifestyle. She was sorry, she told me, but she just could not give up her favorite foods. She left my office, and I did not see her again for two years.

By the time Louise returned, her fibroids had expanded her uterus to a twelve-weeks-pregnancy size. They were causing heavy menstrual bleeding, pressure, cramps, and fatigue, and Louise's doctor was recommending a hysterectomy. Louise was also even more overweight by now. She was finally worried enough about the harmful effects of her weight and the fibroids to consider some healthy changes. She abandoned her SAD eating style and committed to a gradual but definite switch to more healthful foods. She was also willing to follow the other components of a total healing program to help boost her health and shrink her fibroids.

By the end of a year, Louise had dropped twenty-five pounds and her uterus had shrunk to a nine-weeks-pregnancy size. She is still sticking to the diet and losing weight, and she remains symptom-free.

SAD Food Groups

Virtually every holistic and nutritional health expert agrees that certain foods should be avoided altogether because they rob you of health and energy. Let us take a good look at these foods:

SIMPLE SUGARS AND REFINED STARCHES

Simple sugars and refined starches deteriorate health and promote fibroid growth because of the following negative effects:

- Hormone imbalance. Simple sugars and starches are deadly to your overall health, and they wreak absolute havoc on hormone balance. That rush of energy you get after eating a candy bar or glazed doughnut lasts all of fifteen minutes to half an hour. The rush comes from a sharp rise in your blood sugar levels, but that "high" soon switches direction and plummets downward, leaving you drained and exhausted. Over time, the up-down swing pattern leads to a condition called hypoglycemia in which your blood sugar levels are chronically low. You drag through your days feeling depleted, emotionally unstable, and constantly tired. Other possible symptoms of this blood sugar imbalance include daytime panic attacks and waking up in the middle of the night, sweating, heart racing. You are in a state of emergency because your adrenal glands are secreting extra cortisol in order to replenish sugar levels in your system. Sugar is an essential fuel for every system in the body, especially the brain. Over time, this extra secretion stimulated by chronic low blood sugar levels weakens the adrenal glands and leads to hormone imbalance. Why does this happen? The precursor hormone for cortisol is progesterone, and when progesterone becomes overly occupied with producing extra cortisol, less progesterone is available to balance estrogen. A state of estrogen dominance develops—the ideal condition to promote such hormone-imbalance problems as PMS, menopausal difficulties, endometriosis, and fibroids.

• B-vitamin deficiency. Constant cortisol secretion caused by a high sugar/refined carbohydrate diet also impairs hormone balance another way. By keeping your body in a chronic state of alert, continuously poised for fight or flight, you use up the same nutrients you need for proper hormone balance and optimum general health: the B vitamins, especially B_6, as well as magnesium.

The sugar blues do not end here.

• Syndrome X and type 2 diabetes. In order to get all this sugar out of the blood and into cells, where it is converted into energy, the pancreas has to keep secreting insulin. If too much blood sugar stimulates excess insulin secretion, insulin receptor sites become less responsive to that hormone. This condition is called insulin resistance, and it means that more and more insulin needs to be secreted in order for that hormone to enter enough receptor sites and provide cells with the fuel they need in order to produce energy. When the blood is loaded with excess insulin, you have a condition called Syndrome X. People in the alternative health field have long recognized Syndrome X, but conventional medicine only recently acknowledged it. Syndrome X is characterized by a complex disease picture: elevated triglycerides (a form of fat in the blood that is a risk factor for cardiovascular disease in women), obesity, hypertension (high blood pressure), and blood sugar levels so elevated that they eventually lead to adult-onset-type diabetes.

Here is how elevated insulin levels affect fibroid conditions: those high blood levels of insulin also reduce the levels of a protein in the blood called sex-hormone-binding globulin (SHBG). SHBG transports most of the estrogen in the bloodstream. SHBG attaches to estrogen, making excess estrogen unavailable to the estrogen receptor sites on the cell membranes. In this way, SHBG helps prevent estrogen-dominant states. In fact, SHBG is supposed to bind over 90 percent of circulating hormones to keep them from over-stimulating the hormone receptor sites. Only free estrogen, the estrogen that is not bound to SHBG, can dock on a receptor site and form the hormone-receptor-site complex that creates changes in the body. When too much sugar is consumed and insulin levels rise, levels of SHBG decrease, allowing more free estrogen to get into cells. Too many receptor sites become stimulated, which results in the estrogen-dominant state associated with the development and growth of fibroids. And that's *still* not the entire sad story on sugar!

- Compromised immune response. Contrary to popular wisdom, a spoonful of sugar does not help the medicine go down. Studies prove quite the opposite: just a single teaspoon of sugar reduces a child's immunity for up to four hours after it's consumed.
- Raised cholesterol levels. Elevated sugar levels in the blood cause cholesterol levels to rise also. Cholesterol is a hormone precursor, which means that it is used to make hormones. When cholesterol levels rise, estrogen levels in the blood become higher as well.
- Yeast infections. More and more people are now realizing

that the troublesome yeast infections, like *Candida albicans,* that afflict so many women thrive on diets heavy in sugar. Yeast infections do more than cause annoying and recurrent vaginal problems. If they are serious enough, these infections also compromise healthy intestinal function. An unhealthy intestinal tract overrun with yeast organisms does not allow for optimal elimination of hormonal wastes, which can be a major cause of excess levels of estrogen in the body. Yeast also creates a mycotoxin that seems to have strong estrogen-like effects, further increasing the hormone imbalance.

Understanding Dietary Fats

A lot of confusion clouds the truths about the controversial subject of dietary fats. In our Barbie Doll "thin at any cost" society, *all* fats have been slapped with a bad reputation. The truth is all fats are not bad, and "fat-free" usually means chock-full of sugar. The problems with fat come only from eating the *wrong type of fat.*

We need certain fats for optimal health and hormone balance. The right fats help us absorb and store proper amounts of fat-soluble vitamins A, D, E, and K, all of which are key to smooth organ and gland functioning and peak gynecological health. Fat is also the most concentrated source of body energy, and it is an essential source of energy on the cellular level.

SATURATED FATS

The so-called bad fats are saturated and found mostly in red meat, poultry, dairy products, and also in shellfish. Hydrogenated or partially hydrogenated oils, such as margarine, also known as trans-fatty acids, are thought to be even more threatening to your health. Saturated fats are solid at room temperature, and hydrogenated fats have been chemically altered so that they will become solid at room temperature. Margarine is a good example of a hydrogenated or partially hydrogenated fat that was developed from a liquid fat so it could substitute for butter during World War II. These bad fats wind up taking the place of healthful essential fats in the membranes of the body's cells. Saturated fats comprise all animal fats, which also include lard and milk products. This type of fat contains an essential fatty acid called arachidonic acid, which the body uses to produce the series 2 prostaglandins that promote inflammatory reactions and cramping. This means that a heavy dairy and meat diet will worsen any fibroid-related discomfort.

Excessive amounts of dairy products and animal meat provide fibroids with the perfect fuel to help them flourish and grow. This is especially true if the animal products are not free-range or organic, that is, free of antibiotic, hormone, insecticide, and pesticide residues. All commercial meat and dairy products contain these residues, and their dangerous estrogenic action in the body plays havoc with a susceptible woman's hormone system.

Cows are given anabolic steroids to beef them up—no pun intended. Steroids have even been implanted in chickens during their growth phase. Although breeders claim that the chickens and cows excrete all these steroids, residues are found in their meat, and holistic health experts believe that eating this meat can create steroid-like effects in humans.

Dairy cows are routinely given large doses of antibiotics because they often suffer from mastitis, an infection of their udders and nipples. They are also dosed with insecticides and pesticides through their feed and through having their stalls sprayed for rodents and insects. As if that were not enough, bovine growth hormone (BGH) is given to these cows to increase their milk production. You may have heard of human growth hormone (HGH), used in a controversial antiaging therapy that is widely believed to increase risk for tumors, including breast and prostate cancer and fibroids. Bovine growth hormone is similar. Unfortunately, dairy farmers are not required to indicate if they use bovine growth hormone in milk production. So, unless a milk carton states explicitly that the milk is free of BGH, you cannot be sure whether that hormone is present.

We know that human GH stimulates production of a hormone called insulin-like growth factor (IGF-1). Elevated amounts of IGF-1 are associated with hormone-dependent cancers, such as cancers of the breast and prostate. The descriptive name "growth factor" tells you everything you need to know. This stuff makes things grow. Therefore, women trying to shrink the size of their fibroids would be wise to eliminate or at least cut down on these substances.

Kurt Osler, a physician in Connecticut, has also discovered that bovine xanthine oxidase, an enzyme found in cows, is found in humans who consume homogenized milk products. Bovine xanthine oxidase is known to have harmful oxidizing effects on human tissue. For that reason, it may be responsible for increasing the incidence of arteriosclerosis, or hardening of the arteries.

Milk and dairy products create other problems, especially for fibroid sufferers and small children. Many mothers of young children are not aware of the connection between dairy products and ear infections. Children who are treated over and over with antibiotics for recurrent ear infections often find relief after they are taken off dairy products. It seems that dairy products set up the child for higher risk of infection by increasing mucus production in the ear. The pelvic organs are lined with the same mucous membranes that line the inner ear. *I strongly believe that this is why dairy products pose the same increased risk for congestion in the pelvic area, where they also cause excessive mucus production.*

Dairy products are also a common food allergen that interferes with normal intestinal digestion and elimination in susceptible people. As you already know, an unhealthy digestive tract makes a woman more vulnerable to disorders related to hormonal imbalance.

If you do eat meat and dairy, eating organic dairy and free-range meat is much better, because these animals are allowed to roam freely, and they are not fed grain contaminated with pesticides and insecticides. Eating small amounts of lean range-raised meats will not cause health problems in most people. However, women who have fibroids—or other problems related to hormonal imbalance, such as endometriosis and PMS, where inflammation and/or cramping is common—should avoid meat, at least until their condition is corrected. Again, this is because saturated fat contains arachidonic acid, which causes inflammation and cramping by producing prostaglandin E2. Poultry seems to have the largest amounts of arachidonic acid. Even skinless free-range poultry, or small amounts of lean free-range meat, is not a great idea for women suffering from difficult-to-treat conditions related to hormonal imbalance, such as fibroids.

Here are other related health risks posed by "bad" fats:

• Unhealthy cell membranes. Every cell membrane in the body is composed of fats. These membranes created from fats determine which nutrients and hormones get into the cell and how quickly they enter, so that the cell can do its job. The fats that line the cell membranes also dictate the shape and flexibility of each cell. But cells lined with membranes created by the wrong kinds of fats are too unhealthy to transport essential nutrients into the interior. These cells are also typically inflexible and generally incapable of functioning as they should.

• Thickening of the blood. Cell membrane stiffness can also lead to thickening and "sludging" of the blood, which increases the chances for blood clots, strokes, and heart attacks.

• Impaired circulation. Many circulatory problems are related to poor dietary fat choices that cause red blood cells to become so stiff that they cannot squeeze through the body's small capillaries to make deliveries of oxygen and other essential nutrients to every part of the body. This is especially true for the extremities and other body areas where red blood cells must flow through very narrow capillaries in order to deliver their goods. This condition can lead to a host of serious health problems.

WARNING: If you overheat healthy nonhydrogenated fats (also known as mono and polyunsaturated fats), these "good" fats actually turn into "bad" ones. The high level of heat involved, for instance, in frying alters their chemical structure so that they transform into harmful free radicals that destroy cells. Standards have been established for acceptable amounts of these harmful fats in your diet. Be sure to check food labels to make sure the food contains only low amounts of these fats, but I advise you to avoid them altogether.

THE GOOD FATS

Let us take a look at the two other major types of prostaglandins. The E1 and E3 series are the "good" prostaglandins. They are made from the healthful dietary fats that you want in your diet; they contain the omega-3 and omega-6 essential fatty acids. You get these healthy EFAs from deep-sea cold-water fish. Healthy EFAs are also in such nonhydrogenated oils as flaxseed (the best source), hemp seed, safflower, canola, wheat germ, sesame seed, walnut, olive, and soybean; other nuts and seeds; and organic eggs laid by chickens that eat feed supplemented with the fish oil DHA (docosahexaenoic acid). Good-quality omega-6 fatty acids are easier to get from food: walnut oil, macadamia oil, sesame oil, hazelnut oil, black currant oil, evening primrose oil, borage oil, and most vegetables. Most people are well supplied with the omega-6 fatty acids but deficient in the omega-3 fatty acids. The omega-3s are found most abundantly in flaxseed and deep-sea cold-water fish, salmon, sardines, tuna, halibut, mackerel, and cod.

The body manufactures "good" prostagladins from the omega-3 and -6 essential fatty acids via a transformative chain of events. Omega-6 fatty acids are transformed in the body into GLA, or gamma-linolenic acid, and then into the E1 series of "good" prostaglandins. The E1 series acts like an antispasmodic hormone for the uterus, so it prevents excessive cramping during menstruation. The

E1 series of prostaglandins also reduces PMS symptoms, fibrocystic breast disease, and pain associated with fibroid tumors.

The E3 series prostaglandins are made from a fatty acid called alpha-linolenic acid, which is primarily found in flaxseed, walnuts, and hemp seed. The alpha-linolenic acid is converted in the body into eicosapentaenoic acid (EPA) and docosahexaenoic acid (DHA). EPA and DHA then become the E3 series. EPA and DHA are also found ready-made in deep-sea cold-water fish.

This E3 series of prostaglandins is particularly effective in reducing the painful symptoms of fibroids (and endometriosis) because it produces an anti-inflammatory effect throughout the body. Double-blind placebo-controlled studies also show that the E3 series of prostaglandins is effective in reducing the pain and inflammation associated with conditions such as rheumatoid arthritis. The oils from deep-sea cold-water fish also reduce levels of triglycerides, or "bad" cholesterol, which pose independent risk factors for cardio-vascular disease in women.

Since your body manufactures the E3 series of prostaglandins from the oils of flaxseed and the flesh of deep-sea cold-water fish through a complex series of reactions, this transformation depends on the presence of numerous cofactors. These include a high enough intake of magnesium, vitamin B_6, and zinc.

If you do not consume the right foods to create a balance between the omega-6 and the omega-3 fatty acids, you risk hormone balance disturbance. As I already noted, most of us have too much omega-6 fatty acids and not enough omega-3s. If you are not eating enough foods that contain omega-3s, try to add them to your diet, along with foods that are rich in magnesium, vitamin B_6, and zinc. You may also want to supplement with blended oils or capsules. (I will tell you exactly how to do this in Chapter 5.)

A number of telltale signs can let you know if you are not eating enough foods containing omega-3 fatty acids: dryness of the skin, eyes, and mouth; constant thirst; constipation; excessive ear wax; and cracks on your heels and/or fingertips, especially in cold weather.

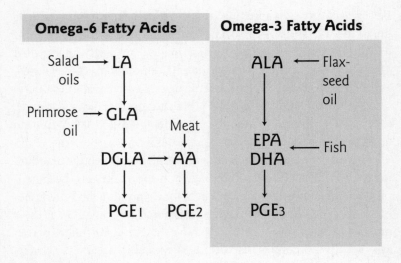

The Fibroid-Healing/Hormone-Balancing Diet

All foods are made up of proteins, fats, and carbohydrates in various proportions. We need all three of these basic elements, but only in high-quality forms. The key to good nutrition is to choose only those food sources that are abundant in quality versions of these elements of life and health. People who live in cultures such as the Mediterranean, where the diet includes fresh fruits, vegetables, nuts, seeds, soy products, grains, and fewer hydrogenated fats, experience far less incidence of heart disease and other chronic diseases associated with aging, such as cancer, diabetes, osteoporosis, and Alzheimer's disease.

They also have a far lower incidence of gynecological problems.

No single diet is perfect for everyone. Some diets stress high amounts of carbohydrates and a low percentage of fats, like the Ornish or Pritikin diets for heart disease, in which 70 percent of the total calorie intake comes from complex carbohydrates. On the other hand, the Atkins diet recommends a high intake of protein and fat, with minimal amounts of carbohydrates. The Paleolithic diet proposed by nutritionist Robert Crayhorn and others stresses high-quality protein and low-starch carbohydrates, because it mimics the diet of our Paleolithic-era ancestors. A similar concept underpins the "ancestral diet," in which you eat the foods consumed by your ancestors in the areas where they originated. In other words, if your family comes from the Slavic countries, your diet would consist of the traditional foods that have been eaten in that part of the world for centuries. The rationale for this diet is that your enzyme system is genetically engineered to deal with these particular foods. A similar line of thinking is behind the diet championed by naturopathic physician Peter D'Adamo and his father, James D'Adamo Sr., N.D., who developed different diets for people of different blood types. Since each blood type evolved during a different anthropologic era, one supposedly should eat the foods consumed during that period in human history. For instance, blood type O is believed to be an old blood type that evolved during a time when people ate animal protein and low-starch-type carbohydrates. The D'Adamos, therefore, recommend that people with O-type blood follow a diet with plenty of lean protein, fish, and greens. Blood type A evolved later on in history, so people with this blood type might do better with more grains in their diet because, at the time blood type A evolved, people were cultivating and eating grains.

The truth is that most people who are generally healthy do well on a diet of high-quality foods that supply anywhere from 30 percent to 55 percent carbohydrates, 25 percent to 40 percent protein, and 20 percent to 30 percent fats.

One point on which most experts agree is that daily fat intake should be kept at 30 percent or less of that day's total calories. The American Heart Association (AHA) recommends a diet rich in grains, fruits, and vegetables, and dictates that total fat intake should be less than 30 percent, with heart-harmful bad fats held at just 10 percent.

It is clear that one diet cannot suit all people, all the time. I developed a hormone-balancing diet for a specific group of women: those who suffer from such hormone-dependent conditions as fibroids. The diet borrows and adapts bits and pieces from other plans to create a total nutritional program that helps the body naturally restore optimum balance. Once hormone balance improves, fibroid growth can be checked, even reversed.

The hormone-balancing diet is a low (animal) fat, high fiber, nutrient dense, vegetarian-style organic foods program that also emphasizes eating plenty of those specific foods known for their hormone-balancing properties. In the past, the diet was vegetarian, but I have discovered that small amounts—generally 3 to 6 ounces per day—of deep-sea cold-water fish such as salmon, sardines, tuna, halibut, mackerel, and herring are health-promoting. I do not recommend dairy products, except for organic, unflavored, unhomogenized yogurt or low-fat organic cottage cheese. I prefer that this yogurt is not homogenized, because the homogenization process preserves some of those bovine enzymes that may be damaging to humans.

MILK SUBSTITUTES

These days we have many excellent dairy substitutes: milk-like products made from soybeans, oats, rice, and almonds can be found in all good health food stores and most supermarkets. Tasty cheese and cream substitutes made from these products are also available.

PROTEIN SOURCES

Women can get high-quality protein from eating a few organically raised eggs per week. I have never seen any evidence to support the claim that eating the entire egg—yolk and white—raises cholesterol levels. Another reason to include whole, organically raised eggs in your diet is that the poultry producing organic eggs is now given feed supplemented with the omega-3 essential fatty acid. This makes their eggs a good source of the essential fatty acid DHA. The amount may not be large, but every little bit of this critical nutrient helps. If your child has been diagnosed with attention deficit disorder or hyperactivity, you should be aware that growing evidence suggests that these children and their breast-feeding mothers are deficient in DHA, which is important to brain and visual development. Evidence further indicates that supplementing DHA can be a key part of the solution and eliminate the need to use powerful and potentially dangerous drugs such as Ritalin.

I recommend that women with fibroid conditions eat at least three servings per week of deep-sea cold-water fish. I do not recommend farm-raised fish, because I am not sure what these farm-raised fish are fed. It could be that they also eat the same pesticide- and insecticide-heavy grains that are given to land animals, or even feed containing animal by-products that could be contaminated with factors responsible for mad cow disease. As I stated earlier, fish from deep, cold oceans also supply a good amount of the essential fish oils that the body uses to manufacture anti-inflammatory E3 prostaglandins. These prostaglandins are helpful to anyone suffering from fibroids and experiencing pelvic pain.

FRUITS AND VEGGIES

Deep-sea cold-water fish are a source of good fats because they feed on algae that is rich in healthy essential fatty acids, so it makes sense for humans also to eat a lot of greens that are high in these helpful essential fats. Like these fish, we need to feed on the garden "weeds" we normally try to get rid of (like purslane, which contains more omega-3 fatty acids than any other green), because they provide us with a healthier balance of essential fatty acids.

So, eat plenty of green, leafy vegetables. Like other foods, your vegetables should be organic, that is, free of pesticides and insecticides, and grown in soil that is rich in nutrients important for optimal health. Most commercial vegetables are grown in soils "enriched" only by a nitrogen-potassium-phosphorus combination (NKP) that gives vegetables the bare minimum of fertilizer to make them look good. Unfortunately, this soil is deficient in important trace minerals such as manganese, zinc, copper, magnesium, selenium, and others crucial to gynecological health. Studies have shown that organically raised vegetables contain higher levels of health-promoting trace minerals.

Cruciferous vegetables like broccoli, cauliflower, cabbage, brussels sprouts, kale, and Swiss chard are standouts for their ability to help metabolize hormones in a beneficial way. Estrogens in the body can take several different paths in order to be excreted from the body. As you know, the liver can change estrogen into beneficial by-products or harmful by-products, depending on the basic chemistry of your body. Cruciferous vegetables contain a number of substances that help estrogen transform into beneficial by-products. These include indole-3-carbinol, which helps estrogen metabolize properly and take a beneficial route out of the body. The more "good" metabolites the liver makes—in other words, the more safely metabolized estrogen—the less the risk of hormone-dependent problems like fibroids. Bad metabolites increase the risk for fibroids, endometriosis, PMS, and other hormone-dependent problems, including various cancers. Eat your broccoli!

Onions and garlic—and their relatives the garlic shoot, leeks, chives, and scallions—help maintain gynecological health because they are potent antioxidants. Antioxidants prevent free-radical damage to body tissue. You know that a piece of iron left out in the rain will rust. The rusting process is similar to what happens in the body whenever tissue is exposed to free radicals. Antioxidants work almost like a protective coating to prevent "rusting" of body tissues. Garlic also contains a factor that prevents the formation of new blood vessels called antiangiogenesis factor. In this way, garlic is important in preventing and shrinking fibroids, because fibroids need many blood vessels in order to grow. Fibroids actually produce a substance to stimulate blood-vessel formation, so the antiangiogenesis factor counters that effect.

Root vegetables—turnips, parsnips, beets, and carrots, to name just several—come in many colors because these vegetables contain bioflavonoids and carotenoids, which are major antioxidants. The bioflavonoids also function as weak estrogens that help to push stronger and more harmful estrogens away from estrogen receptor sites. In addition, they have the unique function in the body of protecting and strengthening small blood vessels. This can be extremely helpful to women with heavy or irregular bleeding due to fragile blood vessels in the uterus.

Vegetables also contain vitamin C, which helps prevent miscarriages. Mounting evidence suggests that this water-soluble vitamin also supports adrenal gland and hormone function. Virtually all vegetables and fruits contain vitamin C, but citrus fruits are particularly rich in this important nutrient.

The bioflavonoids found in some fruits work in your body in tandem with vitamin C. In fact, C and bioflavonoids are often found together, particularly in the white pulp under the skin of citrus fruits. That is why it's best to eat the whole fruit, rather than just the juice, so you can reap the benefits of this nutritional synergy.

Fruits and vegetables provide your safest source of vitamin A. There are two types of A. Retinol comes from animal sources. Carotenoids are found in vegetables and fruits and then converted by the body into vitamin A. Carotenoids are the safe form of this vitamin, because your body cannot create more than 5,000 units of vitamin A from that source. Vitamin A is necessary for optimum hormone production and balance, but commercial food processing robs your food of this key nutrient. On the other hand, this fat-soluble vitamin is stored in the liver. This means that taking a lot of vitamin A, particularly in supplements using the less safe retinol form, while helpful in some situations, can also be toxic. So use high doses only under the supervision of a knowledgeable practitioner.

Root vegetables such as onions, potatoes, carrots, turnips, and yams and leafy green vegetables such as kale and collard greens also contain healthy amounts of calcium, magnesium, phosphorus, zinc, iron, and trace minerals—as long as they are grown organically.

One way to make sure that you are getting your essential nutrients from fruits and vegetables is to eat as many different-colored vegetables and fruits per day as possible. The government's minimum recommended daily allowance (RDA) of fruits and vegetables is five servings per day. These minimum amounts prevent obvious disease. Five fruits and vegetables per day are not enough to create optimal health, and most people do not even come close to that bare minimum! Be sure to eat at least six or more different-colored fruits and vegetables per day, so that you will get a good selection of all the different nutrients they contain. Each bioflavonoid and carotenoid targets a different organ, so a good mixture of colors is essential. I am advising you to eat as many colors as possible, but please do not follow the example of my children, who try to pass off a handful of M&M's as getting all of their colors.

NUTS AND SEEDS

Seeds (especially flax) and nuts are another excellent, highly nutritious food source because they pack high amounts of vitamins and healthy essential fatty acids, and because they are concentrated sources of high-quality non-animal protein. Flaxseeds also contain phytoestrogenic substances called lignans, which help balance estrogen levels by competing for estrogen receptor sites against the body's stronger and potentially harmful natural estrogens, as well as against the even more dangerous xenoestrogens found in chemicals.

I recommend about two to four tablespoons of ground-up flaxseeds daily. Sprinkle them in soups, cereals, and on salads. I like to combine flaxseeds with pumpkin and sunflower seeds to get a more balanced mixture of the essential fats. Since pumpkin seeds are one of the few good sources of zinc, it's a good idea to include them in your regular diet, because zinc is an important mineral for hormone balance. Zinc promotes production of testosterone, the libido-boosting hormone that also keeps the body toned and strong. Another good source of zinc is oysters, which is why oysters have a reputation as an aphrodisiac. Few of us eat enough oysters to get sufficient amounts of hormone-balancing zinc. In fact, many people do not even consume the RDA for zinc.

HEALTHFUL CARBS

We need complex carbohydrates for energy. We have all heard about marathon runners who consume huge servings of pasta the night before a race. But the rest of us who are not marathon runners do not need carbs in such large amounts, and there is a problem associated with carbs, especially for women who are trying to shrink fibroids. Many carbohydrates have what is known as a high glycemic index. This means that the body identifies and reacts to these carbs as if they were pure sugar. As you know, eating too much sugar creates excess insulin production that leads to widespread hormonal imbalance and possible insulin resistance. In order to correct hormone imbalance and stop fibroid growth, avoid any food with a high glycemic index, even if the carb is complex, that is, a whole grain.

Carbohydrate, or starchy, foods with a very high glycemic index include potatoes, yams, sweet potatoes, and flour products, such as pasta, breads, cereals, and pastries. Another problem with commercially grown wheat (barley, rye, and oats) is that the gluten (a protein) is especially powerful these days; many people are sensitive to gluten and experience allergic reactions. In addition, studies show that gluten can interfere with the liver's ability to metabolize estrogen—yet another reason for women with fibroids to avoid high-gluten foods. However, other research indicates that if you add a good-quality fat to a meal that also contains a high-glycemic starch such as pasta, it does not turn into sugar in the body quite as rapidly. You will not get that insulin surge that leads to hormonal imbalance. I recommend adding olive oil to meals that contain such typical complex carbohydrates as potatoes, pasta, or bread.

Nongluten grains, like rices, millet, and buckwheat, are a better choice because they are more alkaline. Fibroid conditions seem to thrive in an acid environment, so adding these alkaline foods to your diet can help prevent their growth. More important, these grains are gluten-free, which means that they are free of the protein in wheat. Oats are also a gluten-containing grain, but many people seem to do well with oats. In my experience, a majority of women who have symptomatic fibroids and are sensitive to gluten are also lactose intolerant, which means they cannot digest milk and other dairy products. Because so many women experience sensitivities to both gluten and dairy, I recommend that those who have symptomatic fibroids use only gluten-free grains and avoid dairy products for at least the first six months of their program. Instead, they eat plenty of brown rice, long grain rice, basmati rice, wild rice, millet, and buckwheat; if they are not sensitive, oats are also fine.

You need these whole grains for their vitamin E (tocopherol complex) content. Vitamin E is popularly known as the sex vitamin, because it affects the reproductive system so profoundly. Vitamin E is an amazingly effective antioxidant, which means that it prevents your body's cells from merging with oxygen or being oxidized, which could then destroy them. Another reason to eat vitamin E–rich foods is its benefit to the pituitary gland, the body's master gland that plays such an important role in maintaining hormone balance. E also prevents excessive blood clotting and helps maintain normal menstrual flow. Many people also find they need to supplement vitamin E because it's difficult to get enough vitamin E from food alone, especially if you are over forty, when your supply of E starts lowering as your need increases. (Chapter 5 gives you guidelines on supplementing this essential nutrient.) It is best to get as much as possible from your food, while still avoiding high-glycemic grains. Other foods containing plenty of E include wheat germ, soybeans, peanuts, asparagus, salmon, spinach, nuts, sunflower seeds, and oils made from sunflower seeds, safflower seeds, almonds, sesame seeds, peanuts, and olives.

Whole grains provide lots of the B vitamins, also known as the energy vitamins, because they are essential for healthy, balanced nervous system function. Without energy and a strong nervous system, your gynecological health suffers. The Bs also boost levels of testosterone, the male sex hormone that is also present in females—although in far lower levels—and is responsible for a healthy libido, good energy, and the drive and ambition to accomplish your daily goals. You must consume adequate amounts of all the Bs, because they work together. Low levels of just one means the others cannot do their job. So eat from a variety of vitamin B–rich foods to maintain and improve gynecological health.

All whole-grain foods contain high levels of B complex vitamins. Again, avoid the grains with a high glycemic index, but eat plenty of alkalinizing grains, such as brown rice, long grain rice, basmati rice, wild rice, millet, buckwheat, and oats.

LEGUMES

You diet should also include legumes—beans and peas. These are good complex carbohydrates that tend to alkalinize rather than acidify the body. Like nuts and seeds, legumes contain the lignans that help balance the body's hormones because they are phytoestrogenic. Again, this means that they act as harmless, mild estrogens so they compete against stronger, more harmful estrogens for the body's hormone receptor sites.

Soy and food products made from soy are phytoestrogenic legumes that should be important components of your diet. Soy contains plant estrogens called isoflavones that also compete with harmful animal estrogens for estrogen receptor sites within the uterus and fibroid tumors. Genistein and daidzein are two soy "estrogens," or isoflavones, that discourage fibroid growth by beating those harmful estrogens to receptor sites. In that way, they help balance hormone levels. Many good soy products can boost your isoflavone consumption. Nearly every morning, I make a breakfast shake containing, among other ingredients, a soy protein powder called UltraMeal, which is available through a mail-order "nutraceutical" company called Metagenics or through licensed doctors, acupuncturists, and chiropractors. I start my day with this shake because soy's health benefits apply to men as well as women, and it is a convenient, time-saving way to pack many essential nutrients into one quick meal. I simply do not have enough time in the morning to meditate, stretch, then sit down to a large, well-balanced breakfast, and still get to work on time. So I developed my shake recipe to make sure I get the nutrients and energy to start my day right. When I told a few patients about it, they loved it as well. I began sharing my recipe with all my patients, and now I am sharing it with you:

✦ HORMONE-BALANCING BREAKFAST SHAKE

Milk substitute (almond milk, rice milk, oat milk, or soy
    milk, used alone or in combination), to desired
    consistency
1 to 2 scoops UltraMeal*
2 to 4 scoops MetaFiber†
2–4 tablespoons freshly ground flaxseeds (sometimes I
    add pumpkin and sunflower seeds for a more
    balanced blend of the essential fatty acids)
Fruit (I use blueberries, strawberries, or any other
    organic fruit. I recommend berries because they are
    the lowest in sugar and the highest in antioxidants
    and bioflavonoids.)
1 tablespoon fatty acids‡

Add all the ingredients to the milk substitute and blend in a blender.

  * UltraMeal contains 17 milligrams of soy isoflavones per serving. I put one serving, which is 2 scoops or tablespoons, in the blender. Some women use only 1 scoop if they experience bloating or if the shake is too thick for their taste.

  † I add 2–4 scoops of a special fiber product called Meta-Fiber (also available from Metagenics). The fiber helps the beneficial bacteria in the digestive system convert the iso-flavones into an easily assimilated form so they can balance hormone levels.

  ‡ I use Udo's Choice. But Barlean's Organic Lignan Flax Oil, Enzymatic Therapy's Doctor's Choice Flax Oil, and the fatty acids put out by Arrowhead Mills and Spectrum Oils are all effective and easily available.

Make sure to take tablets of vitamin E during the day, in order to prevent these oils from becoming rancid in the body. I prefer the dry form of vitamin E that comes with the trace mineral selenium, because E and selenium work together to augment each other's antioxidant activity, and selenium protects against many hormone-dependent cancers. Depending upon your geographic location, you are probably deficient in this important trace mineral.

You do not have to use UltraMeal. If you prefer, you can use another reputable soy or other isoflavone-containing protein powder, such as Genista, created by Dr. Stephen Holt, a researcher into the health benefits of soy. However, other soy products may not be as good for you. I have examined the labels on many different soy protein products and discovered that most are loaded with refined sugar. These should be avoided. Many contain extremely high amounts of soy isoflavones. I imagine the reasoning behind this is that if a small amount of soy is good, a lot should be even better. This may not be true. Studies are suggesting that large amounts of soy isoflavones may be detrimental. The possible risks associated with eating too much soy may have to do with its phytoestrogenic properties. In other words, too many of soy's phytoestrogens, genistein in particular, may cause fibroids to grow. So far, studies have not come up with any definitive conclusions. Most studies show soy's beneficial effect on conditions of estrogen dominance. Studies that raised suspicions about genistein's possible stimulation of growth in hormone-sensitive tissues like fibroids were conducted *in vitro,* which means that they were carried out in test tubes rather than bodies—human or animal. Most complementary and holistic health-care providers are convinced that soy helps prevent estrogen dominance.

However, eating too much soy can cause low thyroid function. As you know, low thyroid function can also interfere with estrogen-progesterone balance. Soy contains phytates, substances also found in grains and spinach that can interfere with mineral absorption. Eating a balanced diet will prevent this. Another possible drawback related to soy products is that they contain protease inhibitors. Proteases are enzymes that break down and help digest proteins. Protease inhibitors could interfere with protein digestion and absorption, but protease inhibitors are also anticarcinogenic, which means that they prevent cancer. Of course, cancer prevention is yet another potential benefit of eating soy.

Again, just because small amounts of a food like soy are good, larger amounts are not necessarily better. Some women who eat soy with every meal soon start complaining about bloating and stomach cramps. Constant soy exposure causes them to develop a soy sensitivity, just as eating too much of any food can cause you to become sensitive to it. The way to avoid developing sensitivities to a food is to vary your diet, including your sources of proteins.

I usually recommend that your soy protein intake not exceed 25 percent of your total daily protein intake. Your total daily protein intake can range anywhere from 50 to 70 grams of total protein a day, depending on your size, level of activity, and other factors. This daily amount of isoflavones basically mimics the daily amount of soy isoflavones consumed in the standard Asian diet. Asian women who eat this traditional way experience a lower incidence of hormone-dependent health problems.

PURE WATER

Pure drinking water is one of the most neglected yet essential components of a healthful diet. Our bodies are approximately 70 percent water, and all our body fluids depend on sufficient water intake in order to flow and function properly. We need water to make our blood, urine, lymph, digestive juices, and sweat. In the Eastern medical traditions, "dryness" in the pelvis, with an associated reduced level of energy flow, is thought to lead to the condition of "stagnation" that helps create fibroids. Constipation, which is so prevalent in our society and such a major contributor to hormone problems, is related, in part, to not drinking enough water. Mineral water is a good choice because, not surprisingly, it is a great source of minerals.

Many experts suggest that we each drink one ounce of water for every two pounds of our body weight each day. That means that a 120-pound woman needs to take in at least 60 ounces of water a day. In other words, do not wait until you are thirsty to drink water. Carry a water bottle wherever you go. (It is also a good idea to always know where the closest bathroom is located!) Be careful with soft plastic water bottles. Studies indicate that the soft plastic gives off plastic-like compounds when heated, even to the temperature of a warm day. These compounds are hormone mimickers that can introduce harmful estrogens into your body and upset your hormone balance. Use harder plastic containers or make sure not to leave your water bottle where it can be heated, such as in your car on a warm summer day. Another option is to carry your water bottle in an insulated bottle protector that keeps out heat. These can be purchased in any home store.

FIBER

Constipation is a major problem for all the reasons we have already discussed. Many women simply do not give themselves enough time in the bathroom to move their bowels. In effect, they train themselves to have less-frequent bowel movements. When I question patients about their bowel movements, most of them tell me that their bowel movements are normal. If I did not question further, I would miss the key point that these women's notion of a normal bowel movement pattern might be as infrequent as two times per week. All of us need to have a bowel movement at least once a day in order to eliminate the wastes we produce. If you think back to images of large city streets during garbage strikes, you have a good idea of how badly a pattern of infrequent bowel movements can pollute your internal environment. Just think of all those garbage bags piled up on top of each other on the sidewalk, waiting to be picked up, their contents often spilling out through tears in the bags. I remember the last garbage strike in New York City, when garbage overflowed from every sidewalk, attracting all types of vermin. I know that I do not want that kind of waste accumulating in my body.

Adequate intake of fiber is a good waste removal solution. Along with adequate water intake, fiber keeps everything flowing regularly. Fiber also works by supplying fuel to the gut that helps beneficial bacteria grow and thrive. These bacteria benefit many bodily functions and, in particular, help maintain hormone balance. You need a good blend of soluble and insoluble fiber to ensure healthy fiber consumption, like the combination in the UltraFiber I put in my breakfast shake. Another way to keep things moving is to consume regular amounts of fruits and vegetables, and be sure to eat some raw. Whole-grain products also contribute beneficial amounts of soluble and insoluble fiber. I recommend at least 30 to 40 grams of high-quality fiber a day. UltraFiber contributes approximately 7 grams of fiber per serving, which translates as two scoops or two tablespoons. If you are not used to consuming large amounts of fiber, start out with smaller amounts and work your way up. Taking too much, too soon, can lead to excess gas, bloating, and diarrhea. Once your body accustoms itself to increasingly higher quantities of fiber, you will eventually work your way up to 30 to 40 grams a day.

Here is an easy-to-follow summary of the information you have received so far, plus a few new tips on how to balance your hormones and shrink fibroids with your food.

Nutritional Tips for Balancing Hormones and Shrinking Fibroids
- Keep food warm. Just as cold temperatures turn water into ice, which is a stagnant condition, cold foods increase both mucous and pelvic congestion in the body. For this reason, I recommend that women with fibroid conditions avoid cold foods.
- Include liberal amounts of fresh fruits and vegetables of different colors, nonglycemic whole grain, and deep-sea cold-water fish.
- Avoid refined, processed, canned, frozen, and precooked foods. Whenever possible, choose unprocessed and organic

whole foods, raised without the use of antibiotics, pesticides, and insecticides.

• Limit shellfish. They contain essential vitamins and minerals, but they are high in cholesterol and as scavengers may contain contaminants, such as mercury, that aggravate hormone imbalance.

• Use only organic yogurt, and milk and cheese substitutes made from organic soybeans, oats, almonds, and rice.

• Avoid drinking tap water. It is full of chemicals and, on occasion, harmful microbes. Be careful not to leave your soft plastic water bottle in hot cars or anywhere else it can heat up during warm weather.

• Limit caffeine to one to two cups per day, organic, if possible. If you drink decaf coffee, make sure that it is water-processed and not chemically decaffeinated.

CRAMP RELIEVER

Most cramps are caused by an estrogen-dominant state. Caffeine aggravates the problem by interfering with the proper metabolism of estrogen. Caffeine also has a negative affect on the pancreas, causing fluctuations in blood sugar levels that can create or aggravate the symptoms of PMS, breast sensitivity, cramps, and symptoms associated with estrogen dominance and fibroids. Black tea, chocolate, colas, and some over-the-counter medications (including some menstrual pain relief formulas) all contain caffeine. Even decaffeinated coffee contains small amounts of methylxanthines (along with other chemicals your body does not need). Methylxanthines belong to the same family of chemicals that includes caffeine!

To wean yourself off coffee and other caffeinated beverages without experiencing uncomfortable withdrawal symptoms, decrease your daily intake gradually. I suggest purchasing two bags of organic coffee beans, one regular and one decaf. Use a coffee grinder to blend equal amounts together. Slowly, over time, increase the amount of decaf organic beans and decrease the regular beans, until you are drinking decaf entirely. That way you avoid the caffeine withdrawal headache and you will not taste the difference. Again, make sure the label of the decaffeinated coffee reads "water-processed."

Or you can drink a good coffee substitute. Ginger tea has similar stimulating and energizing effects. To make ginger tea, grate a few teaspoons of raw gingerroot into a quart of water. Bring almost to a boil—never allow it to boil, as that will destroy its potency—then simmer for ten minutes. Green tea, which has powerful antioxidant properties, is another good substitute for coffee. Recent evidence also suggests that green tea helps promote healthy estrogen balance. It can be found in organic original and decaf forms. The caffeine in the green tea is a reasonable trade-off for the tea's many health benefits, especially since the original version seems to have more healthful constituents. Green tea also slows down the release of carbohydrates into the bloodstream, so it helps prevent the surge in insulin that can interfere with hormone balance.

• Limit alcohol. Women without fibroids or other conditions related to hormone imbalance may drink one glass of red wine, but not every day. Recent studies indicate red wine may help lower cholesterol. However, there are so many other ways to lower cholesterol levels that I do not recommend starting to drink alcohol for that reason. Women with fibroids and other hormone-imbalance conditions should avoid alcohol altogether because of its harmful effects on the liver and metabolism. One way in which the fibroid-healing diet works is by helping the liver detoxify hormones more effectively. By stressing the liver, alcohol impairs estrogen metabolism, thereby creating a state of estrogen dominance.

• Avoid carbonated sodas. They are full of sugar or artificial sweeteners and, sometimes, caffeine. They are also high in phosphates, which interfere with calcium absorption.

• Eliminate white sugar and products made with white sugar. If you must use sweeteners, try fruit juice concentrate or maple syrup. I prefer stevia to all these sweetening options. Stevia is a South American herbal sweetener that does not depend on insulin for its metabolism, so it does not cause the same problems associated with sugar and sugarlike sweeteners. Stevia is also about ten times sweeter than sugar, so a little goes a long way. If you are prone to yeast infections or low blood sugar, eliminate sweeteners altogether.

• Stay away from all saturated fats and cholesterol-rich foods. That includes meats, whole milk products (especially cheese), most baked goods, all fast foods (doughnuts, hot dogs, potato chips, French fries, etcetera), and all fried foods.

• Use only cold-pressed, unrefined, polyunsaturated oils, such as canola, flax, and small amounts of sesame for cooking, or the mono-unsaturated oil, olive oil. Over the long term, these oils can actually help remove the harmful plaque that builds up on blood vessel walls from a diet of saturated fats. Olive oil makes a healthy and tasty dressing for salads and other foods. Flax is another oil that can be used as a salad dressing. You can also experiment with more exotic oils like hazelnut and walnut.

• Never fry foods. Do not heat unsaturated fats to high levels, as heat creates the free radicals that have been implicated in aging diseases of the body and turns good oils and fats to bad. Extract the nutritional benefits from your vegetables either by steaming them lightly or cooking them briefly in the microwave. Stir-frying, using less oil and small amounts of water, is a good way to prepare food. I learned a trick from my wife: stir-fry garlic and onions in small amounts of olive or canola oil, before adding the vegetables. The antioxidant effect of the onion and garlic protects the oil from free radical damage. Broil, pan broil, roast, or bake fish.

• Use salt sparingly—use only sea salt. Using sea salt also ensures sufficient mineral intake, and that type of salt is also a good source of iodine, a mineral that is important to healthy thyroid function and hormone support in general.

• At the same time, avoid processed foods containing large quantities of sodium. Use small amounts of sea salt in the preparation of your food and sprinkle it lightly to taste on your meals. Although you want to keep your body's sodium levels from getting too high, adequate levels of salt do ensure your optimum strength and energy. Use natural herbs, spices, and lemon juice to add further flavor. Avoid commercially packaged seasoning preparations. I prefer sea salts that contain good amounts of iodine, in addition to a nice selection of trace minerals.

• Eat plenty of zinc-rich sunflower, pumpkin, and sesame seeds to support hormone production and balance. Many ancient cultures prized these seeds. The gypsies have been eating pumpkin seeds for centuries to balance hormone levels and maintain healthy gynecological function. The women in ancient Babylonia nibbled all day long on sesame seed and honey confections to increase fertility. Modern-day Frenchwomen snack on the same concoction to boost gynecological health. You can do the same by filling a small plastic bag with seeds, and carrying them wherever you go, so you always have a healthy snack on hand.

• Eat smaller amounts of food more frequently. Eating less food in general prevents obesity and its related health problems. In fact, the only effective and scientifically proven way to increase longevity is to restrict calories. So, it may be wiser to eat less in general than to follow Grandma's advice and "clean your plate."

• Chew your food thoroughly. Chewing your food helps

your body digest nutrients completely and brings out the full, naturally delicious flavor of unrefined natural foods. I like the aphorism that advises, "Nature castigates those who do not masticate."

• Eat in calm. My colleague, John Mizenko, M.D., a Chicago holistic gastroenterologist, says that good digestion depends less on what you eat than whom you eat with. Eat your meals in calm, stress-free settings.

Hormone-Balancing Foods

Help balance your hormone levels and heal fibroids by eating a wide variety of the nutrient-rich foods listed below:

FRUITS

Berries of all kinds, apples, bananas, plums, pineapples, cherries, pears, grapes, avocados, pomegranates, quinces, melons, figs, dates, pears, apricots, peaches, nectarines, oranges, grapefruits, lemons, and limes.

VEGETABLES

Beets, radishes, onions, garlic, cucumbers, celery, artichokes, green beans, peas, asparagus, okra, mushrooms, parsnips, corn, eggplants, broccoli, cauliflower, sprouts, and all green leafy vegetables.

WHOLE GRAINS

All types of whole-grain rice, millet, oats, barley, buckwheat, and cornmeal.

LEGUMES

Lentils, peanuts, black-eyed peas, dried peas, and dried beans— soy, mung, black kidney, red kidney, chick pea (garbanzo), pinto, lima, aduki, great northern, navy, white.

NUTS AND SEEDS

Almonds, cashews, Brazil nuts, walnuts, filberts (hazelnuts), pine nuts, and nut butters; sunflower, pumpkin, sesame, fenugreek, and squash seeds and their seed butters, such as tahini (made from sesame seeds). Flaxseeds are your best choice. You do not need to consume tremendous portions of these foods. Small but frequent servings are best, as these nuts and seeds pack a lot of nutrition. Pound for pound, nuts and seeds also have a lot of calories, but small amounts are satisfying.

ANIMAL PROTEINS

Cold-water, deep-sea fish.

You can make up for the lack of animal protein by eating these tasty grain-legume-nut combinations:

> Rice and beans
> Millet and peas
> Whole-grain bread with tofu (soybean) spread
> Baked beans and whole-grain bread
> Millet pudding
> Millet croquettes
> Low-fat granola and/or nuts and seeds
> Lentil soup with sunflower seeds
> Bean, grain, and nut casseroles
> Soy milk custard with chopped nuts
> Bean spread and whole-grain nongluten bread
> Rice and sesame seeds
> Seed butter spread on whole-grain bread
> Bulgur and bean salad

(See the resource guide for recommended vegetarian cookbooks.)

Fibroid-Healing Meals

The following sample meals give you an idea of the kinds of food combinations that provide the quality nutrition your body needs in order to protect your long-term gynecological health and help to heal your fibroid condition. Remember, whenever possible, eat organic.

BREAKFAST

Some people like to start their day with a glass of juice. A far better idea is to eat the whole fruit so that you get all its nutrients in balanced form. In addition, juice concentrates an overly high amount of fruit sugar that can send your blood sugar levels skyrocketing. If you are hypoglycemic and/or suffer from recurrent yeast infections, eat a fruit that is low in sugar, such as grapefruit or papaya, or skip fruit altogether. I find that most people feel better if they start their day with a good protein, along with some fruit and a healthy fat.

> Orange (vitamin C), banana (riboflavin), papaya (vitamin A and digestive enzymes)
> Whole-grain nongluten cereal with ½ cup milk substitute (zinc, calcium, magnesium, B complex)
> Or
> Whole-grain nongluten bread with a nut or seed butter (calcium, thiamin, zinc, B complex) and a boiled egg a few times a week, or four ounces of broiled or pan-broiled deep-sea cold-water fish (protein, essential fatty acids)
> Or
> Low-fat, nonflavored organic yogurt (calcium/lactobacillus—good bacteria). Eat yogurt if you have a severe and persistent yeast problem.
> Or

Hormone-Balancing Breakfast Shake (see page 102)
One cup only of organic coffee (caffeine boost) or ginger or
green tea, or hot water with lemon

MIDMORNING SNACK
Raw carrots (vitamin A) and celery

LUNCH
Organic garden salad made with dark green leafy greens,
yellow vegetables, red peppers, mushrooms, and any
other raw vegetables (high levels of many vitamins and
minerals). Remember to include plenty of different
colors.
Broiled salmon or tuna (zinc, calcium, thiamin, protein,
"good" fats)
One cup whole cooked grain, such as brown rice, millet, or
buckwheat (B complex), or baked potato (vitamin C)
with olive oil
Fresh peas (niacin)or steamed greens (calcium, vitamin C,
B vitamins)
Fruit

DINNER
Large organic garden salad (vitamins, minerals)
Four ounces fish (zinc, calcium, thiamin, protein, "good"
fats)
One cup cooked whole grain (B complex)
Assorted steamed veggies (several vitamins and minerals)
Fresh fruit (vitamins)

EVENING SNACK
A small handful of homemade dry roasted nuts and seeds
(many minerals, especially zinc and protein)
Figs (potassium, calcium, magnesium, iron)

Or

Mix organic homemade dry roasted seeds and/or nuts in yogurt, along with a few pieces of dried figs.

Be kind to yourself when making changes in your diet. Introduce them gradually, and the process will be easier, even enjoyable. As your taste in food begins to refine, natural and nutritious foods become more delicious, and overprocessed, unhealthful fast foods lose their appeal. Eventually, you will grow more in touch with your body's needs and come to view your appetite for certain foods as your best nutritional guide. The following chapter, Fibroid-Healing Supplements, gives you additional information on how supplements can help you meet your daily nutritional quota and protect your gynecological health.

5

Fibroid-Healing Supplements

No More Quick Fixes

As more and more people become disenchanted with conventional medicine's lack of attention to disease prevention, many of us have turned to nutritional supplements to promote balance and health, including gynecological health. When used correctly, supplements help balance hormones and strengthen organs and glands. They also help restore essential body nutrients that are removed by commercial food processing, lost during storage, or gobbled up by the demands stress places on our bodies.

The SAD program does not provide your essential nutrients because SAD foods are composed of sugar, refined starches, and "bad" fats—what are commonly referred to as empty calories. Your store of valuable nutrients that is needed to carry out essential bodily processes is redirected toward metabolizing these empty foods that do not give back any energy to your body. This is why SAD foods are not really empty and harmless. Over the long run, this way of eating can set you up for serious health problems.

Improving your nutritional intake does not mean sticking to a SAD way of life and making up for nutritional deficiencies with a bunch of vitamin and mineral pills.

Ideally, you would meet your quota of vitamins, minerals, and other essential nutrients through your diet, and never have to down handfuls of pills and concentrated nutritional powders and liquids. On the other hand, this is far from an ideal world, at least nutritionally speaking. It is difficult to get all the nutrients you need without taking nutritional supplements, especially if you are in a state of hormonal imbalance.

Many of us who do follow a fairly healthful diet believe that we are receiving all the necessary vitamins, minerals, and other essential nutrients through our food. Two factors make that nearly impossible: the widespread refining and processing of food, and the significant stresses we are exposed to on a daily basis. We all need to supplement our diets with, at the very least, a good multivitamin-mineral.

Supplements can make up for nutritional insufficiencies caused by modern farming methods and overprocessing of foods, but the most important strategy for protecting your health is switching to organic food sources whenever possible.

Many vitamins and minerals are water soluble, which means that they are not stored in the body's fatty tissues and that the excess is excreted through the body's normal channels of elimination. Therefore, water-soluble vitamins usually do not build to toxic levels. However, there are exceptions to every rule. For example, vitamin B_6, also known as pyridoxine, is ordinarily a very helpful supplement, but one study has suggested that doses greater than 200 milligrams per day may cause a disorder in the hands and feet known as peripheral neuropathy. Symptoms include tingling and loss of sensation in the hands and feet, a condition that may not be reversible.

Water-soluble nutrients can also cause problems if they are taken in such excessive amounts that they overwork the liver, kidneys, and bladder—the major components of the body's detoxification and elimination system. Niacin, also known as vitamin B_3, is a good example. Niacin often effectively overcomes cravings in alcoholics and lowers cholesterol levels, but the person must be monitored carefully in order to avoid liver damage. As I have noted earlier, any disturbance in liver function has an adverse effect on gynecological health, because the liver is the primary organ involved in hormone detoxification and elimination.

Vitamin C is sometimes prescribed in high doses by holistic health practitioners—and most famously by two-time Nobel Prize winner Linus Pauling. But those doses can cause abdominal cramps and diarrhea, as well as irritation of the urogenital system that can become chronic and be mistaken for a urinary tract infection. Holistic doctors determine the appropriate amount for an individual patient by pushing vitamin C intake to what they call "bowel tolerance" level. Bowel tolerance means the point at which the mega-dose of C causes diarrhea. When a patient experiences that symptom, she cuts the dose back to about 75 percent, which is the amount of vitamin C her body needs at the particular time. Most mammals make as much vitamin C as they need in their livers, but humans, one or two other primate species, and guinea pigs do not have the required enzymes to complete the vitamin C manufacture process.

Other supplements are fat soluble, which means that they are stored in the body's fatty tissues and that they are best absorbed when taken with a meal that includes some fat. However, if fat-soluble vitamins are taken in inappropriately large doses over a prolonged period of time, they can build to toxic levels and endanger your health. The fat-soluble vitamins include A, D, E, and K (known as phylloquinone in its natural form). Studies show that excess levels of vitamin A taken for a prolonged period can be toxic to the liver. Furthermore, all of us have individual needs and bodies. What is toxic for your system may not be a problem for someone else. For example, high doses of A, in the 100,000 international units (IU) range, have been shown to reduce mortality and morbidity in children of developing countries who have rubella, also known as German measles. In these cases, high doses of vitamin A that would be excessive for another patient group are appropriate, because 100,000 IU of vitamin A is necessary to treat this specific disease condition. Teenagers afflicted with acne also are able to tolerate high doses of vitamin A, and their condition improves when these levels are sustained for several months. Of course, whenever anyone takes vitamin A in such high doses, their health must be monitored with liver enzyme blood tests and attention paid to symptoms of vitamin A toxicity: joint and muscle aches and pains, headaches, nausea, dry skin, hair loss, low blood sugar, and fatigue. Studies also suggest that pregnant women risk damage to their fetuses if they take doses of vitamin A greater than 10,000 IU a day.

Again, no single supplement is a quick fix or a miracle cure. Beware of any company making such claims for its product in advertisements.

Wild Claims and Much Confusion

The subject of supplements can be daunting. With all the wild and extravagant claims made these days by hundreds of supplement manufacturers, how can you know what you should take? Which supplements really work to ensure overall health and gynecological functions? What is best for you?

Patients often ask me whether or not a particular brand of supplement is okay, and they also want to know which are the right brands to use. Some physicians and nutritionists claim that any multivitamin-mineral will do; that it does not matter whether or not a supplement is "natural." Natural health-care providers disagree. Quality does vary from manufacturer to manufacturer, and there are important guidelines to keep in mind when choosing any vitamin or mineral supplement.

The most important consideration is to choose brands that invest part of their profits into research and product development. Those brands might cost a bit more than the Price Club and Costco labels, but you stand a far greater chance of actually getting what you are paying for with companies that conduct research and continually upgrade their products.

General Multivitamin-Mineral Supplements

A good multivitamin-mineral supplement manufactured by a reputable firm and containing the right combinations at the right dose levels is a good way to keep your vitamin and mineral intake at optimum levels, with minimum effort. All you have to do is pop a pill two to three times a day, usually right after your meals. Unless otherwise specified, most vitamins are best taken with food. There are exceptions, however, and I will point them out as we come to them. Here are some guidelines for choosing a multivitamin-mineral supplement:

- Buy hypoallergenic supplements. Many people are allergic or "sensitive" (a broader term that includes more subtle adverse reactions, which conventional doctors often dismiss or overlook) to the binders and fillers used in many tablets. These include waxes, clays, and dyes. Look for a brand labeled "hypoallergenic," which means it is free of allergenic binders and fillers.

- You get what you pay for. When it comes to multivitamin-mineral supplements, you do get what you pay for. Because some of your money is being plowed back into the company's research and development, supplements from these companies may cost more, but you generally get more for your money. The general rule is the cheaper the supplement, the less effectively it will support your health.

- Do not buy supplements labeled "time-release." These contain clays that slow the absorption in your digestive tract. Even if you notice no adverse reactions at first, repeated exposure over time can cause you to become allergic to the clays. Certain time-release supplements are effective. The best way to know which ones they are is to follow the recommendations of a knowledgeable health-care practitioner.

Niacin poses its own time-release problem. Because evidence

suggests that high doses of niacin can be toxic to the liver, a time-release form of niacin was developed to eliminate the need to take many niacin capsules, several times a day. The manufacturers soon discovered, much to their chagrin, that this time-release niacin caused even more aggressive liver damage than an equal amount of the regular capsules.

• Avoid one-a-day brands. These brands attempt to deliver all the nutrients you may need for a day in one pill or capsule. However, it is unlikely that your body will be able to absorb all these different nutrients at the same time, since many of them have to compete for the same transport mechanisms in order to gain entrance into your cells. When "everything" you need for the day is delivered via the same pill, it is comparable to the chaos at the airport check-in area whenever an airline overbooks a flight. Just as some would-be travelers do not get to fly, some nutrients in a "one-a-day" supplement will not make the trip from your intestines into your bloodstream. So, space out multivitamin-mineral-supplement intake over the day, taking one with each meal. That way, nutrients will be effectively transported from your mouth to the rest of your body.

• Check nutrient sources. Many manufacturers claim their supplement is natural, but a truly natural supplement derives its nutrients from concentrated sources of foods, such as beets or alfalfa. Read labels carefully.

• Watch the dose levels of particular vitamins. Fat-soluble vitamins A, D, E, and K are stored in the body fat, where they can build to toxic levels. Again, with vitamin A, symptoms to watch out for include fatigue, nausea, headaches, dry skin, low blood sugar, joint and muscle pain, liver damage, and hair loss. Remember: you can also overdose on water-soluble vitamins. Check the amounts of each vitamin and mineral provided by the supplement against the recommended doses that follow and/or the recommendations of your natural health-care provider.

• Check the bottle label. On mineral supplement bottles,

look for the amino acids "aspartate," "picolinate," "malate," or "citrate." Experts estimate that as little as 10 percent of most mineral supplements is actually absorbed. A good supplement attaches its mineral components to any of the above in order to • increase absorbability.

• Avoid dolomite and oscal as sources for your calcium. Those terms mean that the calcium comes from ground-up oyster shells. Not only will that calcium not be absorbed well, but it can also be harmful. These supplements may also contain lead, a toxic heavy metal that can interfere with neurological and psychological function in children and can be toxic to your liver, kidneys, and gastrointestinal tract. Test if your calcium tablet is dissolving in your stomach by dropping it into six ounces of vinegar at room temperature. Every few minutes, stir the tablet in the vinegar. If the tablet has not broken up into tiny particles after thirty minutes, find a better source of calcium.

• Never take a heavy-duty vitamin-mineral supplement on an empty stomach or with just a cup of coffee. You risk painful abdominal cramps and nausea, and inhibit your body's ability to absorb the nutrients effectively. Always take supplements either midmeal or within twenty minutes of finishing a meal, unless otherwise directed.

• Do not keep an open bottle of supplements more than six to nine months. Always check expiration dates and discard expired supplements. Keep supplement bottles in the refrigerator, especially if they contain fats or oils.

RECOMMENDED CONTENTS AND AMOUNTS
FOR A MULTIVITAMIN-MINERAL

Vitamin and mineral needs differ with each individual, but the following dose levels fall within the range that will ensure most people's health (higher doses may be appropriate under certain conditions, with supervision):

Vitamins

Vitamin A (palmitate is a good source)	10,000–25,000 IU (international units)

Mixed carotenes   25,000–200,000 IU
(5,000 IU of carotene can be converted to vitamin A in the body. The rest will not have vitamin A effects, so it will not contribute the threat of vitamin A toxicity. Again, the maximum amount of vitamin A recommended during pregnancy or for women who are trying to conceive is 10,000 IU. This pertains only to preformed vitamin A, not to carotene.)

Vitamin D   200–600 IU
(This is an important nutrient if you do not get 20 minutes of sunshine every day.)

Vitamin E   100–800 IU
(Higher amounts may contribute to high blood pressure in susceptible individuals.)

Vitamin C   500–2,000 mg (milligrams)
(Again, the dose depends on your body's specific needs; push your dose to bowel tolerance level.)

Vitamin B_1 (thiamine)   10–150 mg

Vitamin B_2 (riboflavin)   10–30 mg

Vitamin B_3 (niacin)   10–200 mg
(If you are under an experienced health-care practitioner's supervision, you can take higher amounts of niacin. Niacinamide, which is often used instead of niacin, can be taken in doses exceeding 500 mg per day, but only under the care of a qualified health-care practitioner. Inositol hexaniacinate [IHN], or no-flush niacin, can be taken safely in doses as high as 1,500 mg per day, without negative effects. It can also be used instead of niacin.)

Vitamin B_5 (panto-thenic acid)   10–1,000 mg

Vitamin B_6 10–200 mg
(Remember: higher doses of B_6 can increase risk of peripheral

neuropathy, so high doses must be monitored by a health-care practitioner.)

Vitamin B$_{12}$ 50–1,000 mcg (micrograms)
(Most people absorb B$_{12}$ from animal products, but the hormone-balancing diet allows little or no red meat. Supplementation may be needed.)

Folic acid   400–5,000 mcg
(This B vitamin is extremely important to hormone balance and to health in general. Folic acid also helps prevent cardiovascular disease, osteoporosis, Alzheimer's disease, and many forms of cancer, including cervical cancer. It should be taken together with vitamin B$_{12}$.)

Vitamin K (phyllo-   70–140 mcg
quinone)

Minerals

Calcium   800–1,500 mg
(Calcium carbonate is all right for most young people who have adequate amounts of stomach acid, but older women with low levels of stomach acid do better with the citrate, citrate/malate, or the microcrystalline hydroxyapatite forms. Less calcium is needed if forms other than calcium carbonate are used, because they are more absorbable.)

Chromium (picoli-   200–600 mcg
nate form)

Copper (sebacate form)   2–3 mg
(This mineral must be balanced with zinc at a ratio of 2 mg of copper for 30–40 mg of zinc.)

Zinc (picolinate form)   15–40 mg

Iodine   150–225 mcg

Iron   10–30 mg
(Iron should be taken only by menstruating females or those suffering from iron-deficiency anemia. If you do not have either condition, do not take iron, as it can be a powerful damaging oxidant that causes free-radical damage in your body.)

Magnesium (citrate,   300–800 mg
    glycinate, and aspartate forms)

Manganese (picolinate   5–20 mg
    form)

Molybdenum   75–250 mcg

Potassium   90–500 mg
    (Your best sources for this mineral are vegetables and freshly
    squeezed vegetable juices.)

Selenium (sodium   100–400 mcg
    selenite form)

✦ Lisa's SAD Story

The story of a patient called Lisa illustrates clearly how the right vitamin and mineral supplement program can be a powerful tool for healing fibroids. Lisa's three older sisters had all undergone hysterectomies for various gynecological conditions. Now, Lisa was facing her turn in the operating room. Like her sisters, twenty-four-year-old Lisa had taken birth control pills for many years. As a busy single woman, she stuck to a cheap, easy, and strictly "SAD" program, seasoned with liberal amounts of chemical additives.

Lisa was in the midst of studying for her Ph.D. when she came to see me. Motherhood was penciled into her life plan for some time in the distant future, but she was worried that the nagging pressure in her abdomen meant the end of that dream. A visit to her regular gynecologist seemed to have proved her right. Lisa had a fibroid that had already swelled her uterus to the size of a six-weeks pregnancy, but her doctor told her not worry, nothing needed to be done. He advised that birth control pills might help, but she knew that her sisters had gone that route, with no success. Lisa did not want to follow her elder sisters' footsteps, so she came to me, hoping I could help her avoid surgery.

During our interview, Lisa also complained of low energy, difficulty sleeping, cramping pain in her pelvis before and during her menstrual periods, and thinning, dry hair. Those complaints, her poor diet, plus the observations I made during her examination, convinced me that her zinc and magnesium levels were too low. This is a very common problem. As many as 70 percent of American women do not even get the government's recommended daily allowance (RDA) of these two very important minerals. Between the two of them, magnesium and zinc are essential to as many as 500 different necessary bodily reactions. Both are very important for hormone balance.

To confirm my suspicions, I ordered a red blood cell (RBC) mineral evaluation and performed the zinc taste test, a simple evaluation of zinc status performed by having the patient hold in her mouth a very dilute solution of zinc. Zinc is connected to the sense of taste, so if the patient cannot detect zinc's characteristic metallic flavor in this solution, she has a zinc insufficiency. I do not often find it necessary to perform more elaborate vitamin and mineral tests. I am not convinced that tests give as much information as a thorough patient history that carefully takes into account current symptoms, even though they may not seem to relate directly to the fibroid condition.

Within the holistic point of view, all symptoms have direct bearing on the problem, because the intricate hormonal web that impacts so greatly on gynecological health also interconnects just about every body part and its function. Deficiencies and problems in one area inevitably affect other parts.

Lisa was willing to follow the hormone-balancing and fibroid-healing diet. She also needed to boost certain mineral and vitamin levels with a regimen that included extra zinc and magnesium, a high-potency B complex tablet, and a capsule of lipotropic factors. Lipotropic factors consist of a combination of the B vitamins choline and inositol with sulphur-containing amino acids like methionine. This helps prevent fatty buildup in the liver that impedes that organ's ability to perform, including its job of detoxifying hormones.

I also showed Lisa how to perform the zinc taste test herself, so she could monitor her zinc levels and avoid overdosing. I also added 2 mg of copper a day to her supplement program to ensure the right balance between copper and zinc.

Only six months into her healing program, Lisa reported that the sensation of pressure in her abdomen had vanished. An exam revealed that her fibroids had shrunk to the upper limits of a normal-size uterus. In a very brief period of time, Lisa was free of all her complaints and symptoms. She continues to follow her healthy lifestyle and visits my office twice a year for a checkup and reevaluation of her supplement program.

Vitamins and Minerals for Gynecological Health and Hormone Balance

Certain vitamins, minerals, and other nutrients are particularly key to maintaining and restoring gynecological health. You need them in higher than normal levels during times of stress or illness; in the mature years; and if you have been diagnosed with a hormone imbalance–linked condition such as fibroids.

- Essential fatty acids (EFAs). These nutrients are called essential because they are not manufactured by the body, but you still need them. You can receive an adequate amount of EFAs from a healthy diet. But I generally recommend supplementing EFAs whenever you need higher levels of E1- and E3-type prostaglandins in order to promote hormone balance, enhance anti-inflammatory response, and relax cramping uterine muscles. As you learned in the previous chapter, E1 and E3 prostaglandins are made from the EFAs found in fish oils and in flaxseed oil. The EFA in flaxseed is called alpha-linolenic acid (ALA). The EFAs in fish oils are called eicosapentaenoic acid (EPA) and docosahexaenoic acid (DHA). A complex series of interactions in your body converts ALA into EPA and DHA. These two substances are then chemically converted into the prostaglandins that restore hormone balance and relieve symptoms of fibroids. Because many nutritional deficiencies can interfere with these conversions, it is important to eat a well-balanced diet and take the supplements that ensure appropriate conversion of fish oils and flaxseed oil.

I have already told you about the Udo's Choice brand, an especially effective mix of "good" EFAs, and about other equally good brands, including Barlean's Organic Lignan Flax Oil and Enzymatic Therapies' Doctor's Choice Flax Oil. Take one to three tablespoons a day of any of those brands, depending on the severity of your condition. For general maintenance of gynecological health, I recommend one tablespoon a day.

• Vitamin E plus selenium. As I mentioned earlier, whenever you take EFA supplements, it is also a good idea to take a daily tablet of dry vitamin E plus selenium, at a dose of 400 to 800 IU of E and 50 to 100 mcg of selenium. This major antioxidant helps prevent the highly sensitive EFA oils from "turning rancid" in your body and creating more health problems from free-radical damage.

Vitamin E also strengthens the immune system and reduces the risk of heart disease and cancer. There are several forms of vitamin E, including alpha and gamma tocopherols, and each probably helps a different part of the body. We know, for instance, that gamma tocopherol is most effective in heart protection. In addition, vitamin E comes in synthetic and natural forms. The natural form of D-alpha tocopherol is best, but it is also the most expensive form. If cost is a factor, it is all right to use the synthetic vitamin E. It may not be as effective, but it is better than not taking E at all. You also have to choose between the amber capsules and dry versions of vitamin E. I prefer the dry E combined with the trace mineral selenium. Many women are deficient in selenium, which not only helps vitamine E do its job but is also thought to reduce the risk of certain hormone-dependent cancers. The brand I use is manufactured by Meta-genics. (See sources in the resource guide.) It combines 400 IU of dry vitamin E with 50 mcg of selenium. The usual dose is 1 to 2 pills per day. Vitamin E is fat soluble, so do not take high doses for long periods of time. With normal supplementation, the only negative effect is that, for some susceptible people, vitamin E can increase blood pressure.

• Bromelain. Boost the EFAs' anti-inflammatory effect with a tablet of bromelain or another pancreatic enzyme, between meals.

• Quercitin. This is a potent bioflavonoid that I will describe a little later on. It should be taken with bromelain to increase the anti-inflammatory effect. Take 300–500 mg, three times per day, along with one tablet of bromelain (2,000–3,000 milk-clotting units [MCU] per day), on an empty stomach. These two supplements often come together.

• Hormone creams. I sometimes prescribe the use of trans-dermal progesterone creams—a fancy term that simply means that they are applied to the skin—to relieve PMS or menopausal symptoms associated with fibroid conditions. These creams are applied to the breasts, upper chest, underarms, insides of the thighs, palms, or soles of the feet, because these areas contain blood vessels that are closest to the skin surface. This is why some experts say to apply these creams to the areas that blush, where they are more easily absorbed through the skin into the bloodstream. The progesterone in the cream helps restore hormone balance and prevent estrogen-dominant states. Creams on the market supply anywhere from 2 mg to 1,000 mg per ounce. I prefer Progest and Femgest, but others with 400 mg per ounce are equally effective (see the resource guide). Each cream contains about 400 mg per ounce, which is the equivalent of about 20 mg per day or one-quarter teaspoon—the approximate amount a normal ovary would produce during the luteal phase of the menstrual cycle. The creams work effectively and have very few negative effects, if any. Apply the white cream to as wide an area as possible and then rub it in. Check the rate of absorption after the cream has been applied by observing the amount of time it takes for the "tacky" sensation to vanish. If the cream disappears quickly, in less than two minutes, your body needs more than the one-quarter-teaspoon dosage. If it takes more than five minutes for the cream to disappear, your body already has nearly enough progesterone, so your ideal dose is less than one-quarter teaspoon. In very rare cases, some women using the cream become emotionally depressed because progesterone has built up in the fatty tissue under the skin. If you apply the cream correctly, this should not happen. A woman typically uses about one ounce per month, for the first few months, and then half an ounce per month after that. Menstruating women use the cream in the luteal phase, or second half of their cycle. Menopausal women use the cream for three weeks out of every month. Do not use the cream during the fourth week, so progesterone receptor sites can recover their sensitivity.

A word about the "yam scam" seems appropriate here. Manufacturers of creams containing wild yam herb claim that this herb converts in the body to either progesterone or DHEA. But wild yam herb and the actual hormones are totally different substances altogether, and no evidence supports their claims. While it is true that constituents of wild yam can be converted into DHEA and progesterone in the lab, the body has no mechanisms to make this conversion possible. Wild yam is a good herb to support adrenal gland function, but it does not act like DHEA or progesterone in the body.

• Vitamin A (and the carotenes). I recommend 25,000 to 200,000 IU of mixed carotenes per day. Vitamin A and the carotenes, of which beta-carotene is the most popular, are fat-soluble vitamins that are best absorbed when taken with a meal that contains fat. Beta-carotene has the ability to be converted into about 5,000 IU of vitamin A per day. However, it is important to take into account that other substances are required for this conversion to take place, specifically, adequate amounts of active thyroid hormone (triiodothyronine or T3). If you do not have enough T3 in your body, you develop the vitamin A bumps on the backs of your arms that I described in Chapter 3. This rough "chicken skin" indicates that low levels of active thyroid hormone are restricting the conversion of beta-carotene into vitamin A. Remember that you also need about 30 mg of zinc, which is best obtained from your food, in order for carotene to be converted into vitamin A.

The other carotenes your body needs are found in the pigment in fruits and vegetables. In fact, the brilliant colors and hues of autumn leaves that attract so many people to the countryside every year are created by the carotenes in trees. In the body, each type of carotene acts as a major antioxidant to prevent free-radical damage in specific organs. Carotenes also reduce the risk of cancer, especially cervical cancer and precancerous conditions. Vitamin A also boosts the immune system, and its anti-infection properties protect the integrity of all the body's surfaces, including all the mucous surfaces that line the respiratory, gastrointestinal, and reproductive tracts. A study in South Africa showed that 50,000 IU of A per day effectively reduced heavy menstrual bleeding. Vitamin A is also thought to help hormone glands make adequate amounts of progesterone. This is certainly important for women with estrogen dominance and fibroids caused by that hormonal imbalance. Again, pregnant women should not take more than 10,000 IU per day, because of the possible risk to the fetus. Studies come up with conflicting results about vitamin A toxicity. So, until there is more understanding of the problem, pregnant women and women trying to conceive should avoid taking more than 10,000 IU. Beta-carotene and mixed carotenes do not have this adverse effect, but they also do not have exactly the same properties and beneficial effects of vitamin A. In general, never take more than 25,000 IU of vitamin A per day, unless under the supervision of a health-care professional.

• B complex. The B vitamin family is an important source of water-soluble nutrients that help the body produce energy from food. They also maintain a balanced immune system by promoting resistance to infection, and they help heal fibroids by promoting a healthy balance of hormones. In general, the Bs restore energy and well-being, and promote resistance to infection.

The B vitamins should be taken together, but individual Bs can be taken separately in higher amounts for their special benefits. Whenever you take a B vitamin separately—for instance, extra B_6—make sure to take a separate B complex tablet at a different time of the day. If you do not, a large amount of one B can interfere with the action of the other Bs. A 50 mg B complex tablet is sufficient for your general vitamin B needs, and it is especially recommended if you lack energy and have poor resistance to colds and flus. Be sure to check with your doctor first to rule out any medical condition that could be causing your symptoms.

B_1. Also known as thiamine, B_1 is crucial for energy production, detoxification, and maintaining balance within the nervous system. This is why alcoholics who suffer from a mental dysfunction called Wernicke's encephalopathy improve with adequate amounts of vitamin B_1. An appropriate dose of B_1 to promote well-being is 10 to 150 mg per day.

B_2. Also known as riboflavin, B_2 is key for the body's energy production. Together with other Bs, B_2 can help in cases of chronic fatigue. B_2 also helps the body regenerate glutathione, one of the most powerful detoxifiers and cancer-protecting agents. In doses of 400 mg per day, B_2 has also been shown to reduce the incidence and severity of migraine headaches. Many women suffer from menstruation-related migraines, so B_2 can be very helpful in such cases. The average dose for B_2 ranges from 10 to 30 mg per day.

B$_3$. This member of the B family comes in two forms: niacin and niacinamide. Niacin has been proven to be helpful in reducing cholesterol levels. Doses of 1,000 mg per day lower total cholesterol and raise the levels of beneficial HDL cholesterol. You can take up to 4,000 mg of niacin per day for its cholesterol-lowering action. When combined with chromium picolinate, amounts of niacin that are as low as 200 mg per day will have similar beneficial effects, without the uncomfortable flushing of the skin that accompanies higher doses of niacin. However, some people need to take high doses of niacin by itself in order to lower cholesterol levels. One strategy for avoiding the annoying flushing sensation is to take niacin at night. Nutritional biochemist Dr. Jeffrey Bland recommends taking one baby aspirin twenty minutes before taking the niacin. Another choice is to take "no-flush" niacin, or inositol hexaniacinate (IHN), at doses of 500 mg, three times per day. It can achieve the same cholesterol-lowering effect without that troublesome flushing. I test many of the supplement protocols on myself before I recommend them to patients, so I can testify to the discomfort of that otherwise harmless niacin flush, even if it doesn't last long.

Niacinamide helps regulate blood sugar levels when taken at doses ranging from 100 to 500 mg per day. It has also been shown to relieve joint stiffness associated with arthritis, when taken in doses of 250 mg, four to six times a day. Both niacin and, to a lesser extent, niacinamide carry a risk of elevated liver enzymes that indicate possible liver damage. That risk is greatest with niacin and with time-release brands, so avoid those. Inositol hexaniacinate (IHN) and no-flush niacin do not pose this risk.

FOLIC ACID. This B vitamin performs many important roles in the body. It is known to prevent a deformity in fetuses called neural tube defects, and it helps prevent DNA damage, making it an effective anti-cancer agent. When combined with zinc and B$_{12}$, folic acid can reverse and/or prevent cervical dysplasia. It also reduces levels of the dangerous amino acid breakdown by-product homocysteine. Homocysteine has been shown in large amounts to be a major risk factor for cardiovascular disease and osteoporosis. Homocysteine may also be a risk factor for other diseases associated with aging. Recent study results report that folic acid is extremely important for the metabolism of estrogens. When the body does not contain enough folic acid, estrogens cannot be detoxified effectively and excreted as harmless waste products. Instead, they become stronger estrogens that create severe hormonal imbalance, upping the risk for fibroids and other hormone-dependent problems. Taking large amounts of folic acid poses no risks. I routinely prescribe 10 mg per day for at least one to two months to my patients with cervical dysplasia. Whenever a patient presents her prescription at the drugstore, I can count on a phone call from a concerned pharmacist who is questioning this high amount. I always reassure them by saying that folic acid is toxic only if you use it to fill your bathtub, then hold your head under the liquid until you drown. The only exception in this case is those people susceptible to a rare form of anemia related to B_{12} deficiency. In such instances, folic acid could mask the symptoms of this underlying problem. Therefore, it is good idea to supplement with small amounts of B_{12}—in the range of 500 mcg per day—whenever you take large amounts of folic acid.

PANTOTHENIC ACID. Also known as vitamin B_5 pantothenic acid works with the other Bs to raise energy levels and maintain adrenal gland health. Overstressed adrenals lead to imbalance in hormone levels and impair your ability to cope with the normal stresses of life. Just 500 mg of B_5, taken three times per day, will rejuvenate the adrenals. Pantothine, an expensive derivative of B_5, is also effective in reducing cholesterol. Take 300 mg, three times a day.

VITAMIN B_6. Vitamin B_6 helps the liver break down estrogen into less problematic metabolites, so the stronger and possibly carcinogenic metabolites will not build to excessive levels and create hormone balance–related problems like fibroids. Vitamin B_6 also helps modulate the effect of estrogens at the receptor site of each cell. B_6 also relieves water retention and breast tenderness before and during menstrual periods and in women with fibroid symptoms. In addition, this B vitamin works closely with magnesium to help produce the anti-inflammatory, antispasmodic prostaglandins E1 and E3. Take either 200 mg of B_6 or 50 mg of the activated form, pyridoxal-5-phosphate (P5P), per day. Do not take more than 200 mg of B_6, unless you are under the supervision of a knowledgeable health-care practitioner. Higher doses could be associated with damage to the sensory nerves, leaving you with numbness and tingling in the hands and feet.

B_{12}. As I told you earlier, B_{12} works with folic acid to maintain healthy DNA. In doses of 1,000 mcg, it also affects mood and cognition. Traditionally, B_{12} was administered by intramuscular injection, but newer sublingual and intranasal preparations are also effective. Since B_{12} is found mostly in meat products, vegetarians must make sure to eat sea vegetables like dulse and wakimi, which also contain B_{12}. They may also have to take B_{12} as a supplement.

• Vitamin C. This vitamin is one of the most widely studied and important water-soluble antioxidants, as it plays many key roles in your body, including protecting other vitamins from free-radical damage, acting as a major anti-infection agent, and protecting connective tissue throughout the body. Vitamin C deficiencies lead to the condition known as scurvy, in which connective tissue breaks down, causing bleeding gums; problems with muscles, the heart, and joints; and eventually, death. During the 1700s, British sailors died from scurvy until it was discovered that eating limes prevented the disease—hence their name Limeys.

Vitamin C is crucial for women with fibroids because it strengthens small blood vessels that can be damaged by heavy bleeding. Even when taken on its own, this supplement can cut back menstrual flow, which may help avoid fibroid-related surgery. Also, by promoting the integrity of connective tissue between cells, vitamin C can make it more difficult for tumors like uterine fibroids to develop in the first place and to grow. The newest facial creams contain high levels of vitamin C to help aging skins speed up collagen repair so elasticity is improved and wrinkling and sagging countered. That should give you a sense of vitamin C's benefits to organ and gland tissue. Doses from 1 to 3 gm per day are enough for most people. But your need for vitamin C can increase during stressful situations, when you should increase your dose up to your bowel tolerance. Again, bowel tolerance means that when you reach a dose level that causes diarrhea, cut back to about 75 percent of that amount. That will be your body's need at that time. Another sign that you are taking too much vitamin C is if you experience irritation when urinating. Again, cut back your dose to a more comfortable level. Of course, this factor makes vitamin C a good antidote to constipation.

Bioflavonoids are often found working alongside vitamin C. Hesperidin and rutin are two bioflavonoids found with vitamin C in the rind of citrus fruit. Isoflavones are found in soy and flaxseed. Quercitin, a powerful bioflavonoid, is found in onions. Proanthocyanidins, contained in grape seed and maritime pine bark, are major anti-inflammatory agents and immune system enhancers that neutralize free radicals in the body and help create hormone balance. This makes them effective weapons against fibroid conditions. Green tea, red wine, and spices like turmeric, thyme, rosemary, and cayenne owe their abilities to balance hormones and reduce abnormally high bleeding associated with fibroids to their high content of bioflavonoids. Take 500 to 1,000 mg of bioflavonoids twice a day, to reduce bleeding and balance hormones. Some practitioners recommend a one-to-two ratio of bioflavonoids to vitamin C.

- Magnesium. A great muscle relaxant, magnesium relieves cramping of the uterus and other symptoms of fibroids, PMS, and menopause. Magnesium is also involved in hundreds of bodily reactions. It helps the liver detoxify hormones, especially estrogens, and participates in forming "good" prostaglandins. It is also prevents and treats osteoporosis, helps heart function, stabilizes blood sugar, and relieves nervous tension. Many health-care practitioners recommend taking magnesium with calcium, at a ratio of two parts calcium to one part magnesium. However, others suggest that the ratio should be closer to one to one. You probably have your own particular need for each mineral, which means there is a ratio of calcium to magnesium that is ideal for you. Most supplements already come in a two-to-one ratio. If your health-care practitioner determines that you need more magnesium, you can add more as a separate supplement.

Some symptoms will let you know if you need more magnesium. If you suffer from chronic cramping, take an extra 100 mg of magnesium glycinate (a well-absorbed form) or aspartate or citrate, every two hours at the first sign of cramps, and make sure you are getting adequate levels of this important mineral throughout the month. As Dr. Jonathan Wright in Washington State says, "If it spasms, give it magnesium." The standard supplement dose is 1,000 mg of calcium to 500 mg of magnesium, taken at bedtime.

- Zinc. Zinc is equally essential to peak gynecological function. Like magnesium, zinc is involved in hundreds of bodily reactions, and, as with magnesium, most people do not even get the minimum RDA from their diets. Zinc is important for the healthy growth of all body tissue and essential for DNA repair. That makes it an important natural cancer-fighting weapon. It helps prevent and treat fibroids because it also plays an important role in hormone production and balance. Since many other nutrients can interfere with zinc absorption, it is a good idea to take a zinc supplement by itself, apart from your other supplements. Some suggest taking it on an empty stomach at night. I test for zinc deficiency with the zinc taste test described earlier in this chapter. Most people need from 30 to 60 mg of zinc per day. Remember to balance zinc with copper, at a ratio of 2 mg of copper for every 30–40 mg of zinc.

CHRONIC INFLAMMATION REMEDY

A combined dose of vitamin E and flaxseed oil can help ease inflammation, including the inflammation that often accompanies fibroids. Take one tablespoon of flaxseed oil and 400 IU of vitamin E every day. When cramping occurs, try taking 500 mg of bromelain, two to three times a day, between meals. This works well with the bioflavonoid quercitin. A good combo for cramps and inflammation of any kind is 500 mg each of bromelain and quercitin, combined with the herb turmeric, taken two to three times a day, between meals.

• Glutathione. Glutathione is a powerful antioxidant, as effective as vitamins C, E, and beta-carotene, but not as popular. Boosting blood levels of glutathione gives you greater vitality. It also naturally detoxifies the body from environmental and bodily toxins that accumulate in the fatty deposits cushioning organs and glands, including those related to gynecological function. Some experts say that glutathione is difficult to absorb when taken by mouth. You can also use other supplements, such as lipoic acid, N-acetyl cysteine, and vitamin C to help your body regenerate its own glutathione. These same supplements also help glutathione promote hormone balance and metabolism.

• Indole-3-carbinol. This chemical, found in cruciferous vegetables such as broccoli and brussels sprouts, helps estrogens convert into healthy metabolites. Besides eating plenty of those vegetables, you can take indole-3-carbinol as a supplement to reduce the levels of strong, potentially dangerous estrogen metabolites. Take 200 mg two times a day.

The detoxification of estrogens occurs primarily in the liver, breast tissue, intestinal tract, and other areas in the body that pitch in with the detoxification process. Fat-soluble substances in the body that need to be excreted are first turned into water-soluble substances so they can be eliminated in the urine and the stool. In the process of making that conversion, intermediary substances are formed that can be more toxic than the original substance. Estrogen is initially converted into the catechol or hydroxy estrogens. There are several varieties of these intermediary estrogens. Some are considered good and others are bad. The good metabolites are the 2-hydroxy (OH) estrogens. These balance the effects of too much estrogen in the body. The bad metabolites are the 16 alpha hydroxy (OH) and the 4-hydroxy (OH) estrogens. These metabolites can actually increase the risk of all hormone-dependent problems, including cervical dysplasia (abnormal Pap smears); breast, ovarian, and uterine cancer; endometriosis; and fibroid tumors of the uterus. They increase the risk of these diseases by their strong and prolonged estrogenic effects on susceptible tissues. But, as with all hormones in the body, there needs to be balance between the good and the bad.

Clinicians can now measure 2-OH and 16 alpha OH estrogens, determine the ratio between them, and take steps to restore any imbalance. Indole-3-carbinol helps the body's detoxification systems increase the production of the 2-OH estrogen. In that way, it helps restore proper balance between the two estrogen metabolites and offset the potentially strong estrogenic effect of the 16 alpha OH and the 4 OH estrogens, thus preventing estrogen dominance that can develop from an abnormal ratio. The Great Smokies Lab and Metametrix Lab test this ratio quite easily in urine or blood. (See the resource guide.)

Other substances that help promote the healthy ratio of these breakdown products are green tea extract, the herb milk thistle, the triterpene D-limonene, flavonoids like lycopene, and all of the nutrients associated with the successful detoxification of homocysteine discussed in previous chapters.

• Calcium-D-glucarate. This nutrient has been shown to reduce the enzyme called beta-glucuronidase, produced in the gut by pathogenic bacteria. As we've said, this enzyme will increase the body's burden of estrogens by reintroducing back into the body estrogens that were supposed to be eliminated. Calcium-D-glucarate is nontoxic and, at doses of 500 to 1,000 mg per day, is very effective in reducing beta-glucuronidase levels until balance is restored in the intestinal environment.

All the supplement products I recommend above can be found at health food stores or ordered through catalogs and Internet Web sites (see the resource guide).

6

Fibroid-Healing Herbs

Nature's Cupboard

The use of strengthening and healing plants is the oldest form of medicine known to man. We know that herbal medicine was practiced as far back as Babylonian, even Sumerian, times. Through the centuries, traditional healers' experiments with flowers, weeds, plants, roots, leaves, berries, and seeds have resulted in a vast stock of natural medicines. These herbal remedies prevent and heal many ailments, and with far fewer harmful effects than those caused by modern pharmaceuticals.

The advent of twentieth-century vaccines, antibiotics, and other pharmaceuticals cast the science of healing herbs into the shadows. That is, until recently. Awareness of the dangers that often accompany the quick fix promised by some modern drugs has increased. As a result, many of us are exploring natural preventive and curative methods that boost the body's own defenses against disease, strengthen overall health and body function, and promote hormonal balance.

Today, we not only have traditional herbal teas and fluid extracts, we can even take botanical supplements in the convenient form of tablets and capsules.

Benjamin Franklin once said, "An ounce of prevention is worth a pound of cure." Plant remedies—prepared as teas, decoctions, tinctures (fluid extracts), tablets, or capsules—deliver powerful protection for gynecological health.

Still, less than 1 percent of the 250,000-odd plant species on earth has been studied for medicinal properties, and many of those valuable plants are being destroyed on a daily basis. Studies to verify the healing powers of herbs cost many millions of dollars. What drug company would underwrite such high costs to verify the strengthening and healing properties of a substance that grows wild—a substance they cannot patent and sell for profit?

Because there is little profit in expensive, double-blind studies for herbs that often grow as profusely as weeds, we mostly rely on anecdotal clinical evidence. Today's holistic health practitioners take into account the reports of other modern-day natural practitioners together with the records handed down from ancient healers to guide our use of healing herbs. Recently, evidence based on research and clinical studies is adding the weight of scientific credibility to what we already knew.

All the evidence supports the contention made by millions of people that nature's cupboard overflows with valuable plant remedies that can help you achieve optimum health, balance your hormones, and shrink fibroid tumors. The path to the peak health and sense of well-being you desire is strewn with roots, leaves, barks, weeds, mushrooms, berries, and even flowers.

✦ Jennifer's Story

A forty-seven-year-old diabetic named Jennifer avoided a trip to the emergency room with the help of two humble herbs. Jennifer had known about her fibroids for many years. They had never given her much trouble, but as she approached menopause, her periods became heavier than ever. Not long after her first visit to me, Jennifer called one afternoon to say that she was hemorrhaging. She had soaked through one sanitary pad in thirty minutes, and the bleeding was getting worse.

Luckily, Jennifer lived near a health food store, so she could easily obtain yarrow and shepherd's purse, two herbs that I recommended she use immediately. I told Jennifer to take one full dropper of a fluid extract made from each herb, every fifteen to thirty minutes. After she took her second dose, Jennifer called again to say she was still bleeding just as profusely. We decided that she would try one or two more doses before going to the emergency room.

Several more hours passed without a word from Jennifer. I was concerned, so I called her. She told me that after her third herbal dose, the bleeding stopped as abruptly as if she'd thrown an "off" switch. Jennifer did not have to go to the emergency room, and her subsequent commitment to a complete fibroid-healing program ensured that she also stayed out of the operating room!

Not everyone's herbal experience is as dramatic as Jennifer's. Most of the herbs I recommend are equally effective, but they work gradually and over a longer term. They help heal fibroids by encouraging hormone balance, toning organs and glands, clearing away toxicity, and relieving congestion in the uterus. All are readily available at health food and herb stores and through mail order. (See the resource guide.)

Until recently, if you wanted to use herbs to improve your health, you had to brew the remedies yourself. Though it can be great fun to experiment with your own remedies, convenience is usually an issue. With many excellent companies putting out herbal preparations of single herbs and compound remedies that make use of two or more herbs working together for a potent effect, you no longer have to make them from scratch.

Types of Herbal Remedies

Whether you purchase your herbs at a store or through mail order or decide to try your hand as an herbalist, use the following instructions as your guide.

BASIC TEA (OR INFUSION) RECIPE

An infusion is a tea made from the leaves and flowers of herbs or from certain berries. Always use pure spring water, distilled water, or filtered water. Bring the water to a boil, then pour the water over the herb. Allow it to steep in a covered container for five to ten minutes. The standard formula for a basic tea is one teaspoon of dried herb to one cup of boiling water, although you might use less herb if it is very strong, more if it is weak. If you are using green (fresh) herbs, use half an ounce of herb to one pint of boiling water. Remember: when making a tea, never boil the herb with the water, as boiling can rob herbal flowers and leaves of their medicinal properties.

Strain out the herbs, and drink while warm. (If you prefer a sweeter-tasting tea, add half a teaspoon of either cardamom powder or licorice root powder to the herb and steep together. You will not need to do this if fennel or licorice is part of a compound tonic. They are natural herbal sweeteners.) Commercially prepared teas are obviously not as strong as those you make from your own herbs. I do recommend the Alvita or the Select brands of herbal tea because they are fresh and therefore effective. The usual dose for a tea is two to four cups a day.

DECOCTION

A decoction is a tea made with barks, roots, branches, and certain berries. It is more difficult to extract the active ingredients from barks, roots, branches, and tougher berries, so you do boil the herbal materials in water to extract their medicinal properties, for ten to thirty minutes. The longer the herbal materials boil, the more medicinal properties you extract. However, boiling time really depends on which herbal ingredients you are using. Again, strain out the boiled plant parts before drinking. The usual dose for a decoction is also two to four cups a day.

FLUID EXTRACTS (TINCTURES)

These are stronger forms of herbal remedies, and there are many fine commercial brands of tinctures or extracts. If you want to make your own, follow these instructions: Chop the herb finely and add one ounce of herb to 1 pint of lab-proof alcohol, which is available in some pharmacies (DO NOT use rubbing alcohol!) or vodka. I recommend using vodka. Shake daily. After two weeks, strain, and use according to instructions. The usual dose is 1 teaspoonful or thirty to forty drops diluted in half a cup of warm water, two to three times a day. If you prefer, you can take it straight. I like to take echinacea straight. That herb is most potent when you experience a characteristic sting on your tongue, and you do not get that sting if you dilute it. My friend Steve Morris, who is a naturopath based in Washington State, makes the most potent echinacea I have ever tasted. If you buy commercially prepared tinctures (also known as fluid extracts), you can follow the dose instructions on the bottle label. I have used and recommend Gaia Herbs, Eclectic Institute, and Herb Pharm.

CAPSULES

Almost any herb can be powdered and placed in a capsule. Of course, it is far more convenient to purchase the capsules, but you can powder herbs yourself—even using a mortar and pestle like the herbalists of centuries ago. All you need is the time and inclination. Once the material is ground down to a fine powder, place it in capsules. The standard capsule size is referred to as "00." Capsules are sometimes not as strong as tinctures or extracts, but they do allow you mobility. Reputable companies are constantly discovering new ways to deliver quality herbs to the public in easy-to-take and effective forms. You can swallow capsules with water wherever you are, and you also have the option of opening the capsules, pouring out the contents, and adding hot water to make a tea. The usual capsule dose is two capsules, twice a day. Again, dose also depends on the herb, so follow the instructions on the bottle label.

Some herbs are standardized to contain specific amounts of their active, that is, healing, ingredient. Remember that modern scientific herbal research is still in its infancy, so we sometimes do not actually know which part of the herb is the active ingredient. For this reason, many herbalists advise taking the whole herb, instead of taking a brand that attempts to isolate what they believe is the active component. For example, it was recently discovered the supposed active, or healing, ingredient of the popular herb Saint-John's-wort is not hypericin, as was previously thought, but hyperfolin. This discovery meant that herbal formulas had to be changed to contain a standardized amount of hyperfolin. Who knew? They may discover that there is yet another active ingredient in Saint-John's-wort that has been overlooked or that you need all the components of that herb working together in order to get the desired effect.

We can be sure that other misconceptions and mysteries have yet to be cleared by the scientists engaged in a quest to discover the active healing principles of various herbs. This is why I stress the importance of buying herbal products from reputable companies that conduct their own ongoing research (see the appendix) and avoiding such brands as Price Club, GNC, and Costco.

GENERAL GUIDELINES FOR MAKING YOUR OWN REMEDIES

Most of the women I work with take herbs in the form of commercially prepared teas, capsules, or tinctures (extracts). A few have found the science of herbs so intriguing, that they learned how to make their own preparations. If you are a budding herbalist, here are the basic instructions for preparing your own remedies:

- If you are able to gather the fresh herb yourself, try to use it immediately.
- Buy dried herbs, or dry them yourself in tightly sealed glass or ceramic containers. Either way, the container will help preserve freshness.
- Always use pure water and organic ingredients.
- Do not use aluminum wares for making any herbal preparations. Aluminum pots and utensils leach aluminum into the preparation, which can cause stomach ulcers. You also increase

the risk of developing aluminum toxicity, which some health professionals believe leads to Alzheimer's disease, osteoporosis, and other health problems. Enamel, glass, and stainless steel pots are best.

PRINCIPLES OF HERBAL HEALING

Though herbs are safer than pharmaceutical drugs, if you want to receive their full strengthening and healing benefits, follow these basic healing principles:

- Different herbs are best used during specific times of the year, especially if you live in a temperate climate. For general use, roots and barks are considered more appropriate to take in wintertime, while leaves and flowers are usually best taken during summertime.
- Dry herbs should not be used after one year, as they lose 50 percent of their effectiveness, even if you picked and dried them yourself. Roots, barks, and some berries can be kept and used longer than most leaves.
- Follow the general recommendation to take herbs at least thirty minutes before eating or two hours after a meal, unless specifically instructed otherwise or if you experience digestive upset after taking an herb. In such cases, take it with a small amount of food that contains fat.
- Unless specifically indicated otherwise, women should not take herbs during pregnancy. Although some herbs are safe during pregnancy, it is always wise to consult first with an expert.

Types of Herbs

Tonic herbs revive energy and stimulate function with a modulating and strengthening action that brings the body, and whatever organ system the herb specifically affects, back into balance. *Nutritive* herbs soothe, calm, and build. *Carminative* herbs expel gas, stimulate stomach secretions, and soothe the stomach muscles and intestinal tract. They also help the stomach absorb and assimilate nutrients and move materials through the gastrointestinal system. *Astringent* herbs help the body absorb fluids, which makes them particularly effective in cases of excess bleeding and diarrhea, both of which are associated with fibroid conditions. *Alterative* herbs, also known as blood cleansers, cleanse, eliminate, and break down excess matter, such the matter that can congest the pelvis, particularly in fibroid conditions. Many herbs in the above categories also contain properties that are antibacterial, antiviral, antifungal, antiparasitic, and anti-inflammatory.

In order to prevent and heal fibroids and other gynecological ailments, your best bets are uterine tonic herbs that promote hormone balance by strengthening and stimulating the adrenals and other glands and organs.

TONIC HERBS

Uterine tonic herbs are generally nontoxic—the safest of all herbs—so they are usually taken over the long term. They can be ingested either individually or in compound remedies that include several herbs working together to strengthen and tone. Tonics can be consumed in many forms—capsule, tincture (extract), decoction, or as an infusion or tea.

Black cohosh (Cimicifuga racemosa)

Also known as squaw root, this popular traditional Native American herb was used by tribal women to speed up childbirth. Black cohosh tends to have an estriol-like effect in the body by lowering levels of LH, or luteinizing hormone. Estriol is the weakest of the three types of natural human estrogens, which is why it does not seem to stimulate the uterus and the breasts as do estrone and estradiol—the strongest natural estrogens. Estriol is also less likely to lead to an estrogen-dominant state that allows fibroids to develop and grow. Studies conducted on menopausal women show that when estriol is given alone, with progesterone supplementation, it does not stimulate the lining of the uterus to grow and thicken. This suggests that estriol will not stimulate fibroid growth either.

Black cohosh helps relieve other gynecological complaints, including menopausal symptoms, and it is considered safe over the long term. All this makes the herb especially helpful to older fibroid patients who need an effective but safe way to relieve menopausal symptoms without risking fibroid growth.

Dose: For a tea, boil two teaspoons of dried roots in one pint of water. Take two or three teaspoonfuls, six times a day. Or take five to thirty drops of the fluid extract in one cup water once a day; or two to three capsules a day. I like the Metagenics version, Black Cohosh Plus, in a dose of one to two capsules, two times a day.

Safety issues: Do not use if you are pregnant or breast-feeding. Very large doses can cause headaches, nausea, abdominal pain, and dizziness.

Borage (Borago officinalis)

Borage leaves are a rich source of calcium and potassium, two minerals important to the nervous system and for calming and strengthening the heart. Borage also tones and stimulates the adrenal glands, which means that it helps promote hormone balance. I recommend borage oil, because it contains the highest amounts of gamma-linolenic acid (GLA). GLA helps your body form the beneficial prostaglandins that reduce inflammation and cramping. It also helps dilate blood vessels so improved blood flow can remove toxins from the pelvic area more efficiently.

Dose: Follow instructions on the label for borage oil. I recommend 250 mg of GLA a day. Other good sources of GLA include evening primrose oil and black currant seed oil.

Safety issues: I do not recommend the use of borage during pregnancy or while breast-feeding, since borage may contain small amounts of liver toxins called pyrrolizidine alkaloids (PA). I do recommend borage products that are labeled "PA free."

Chamomile (Matricaria recutita)

Known for its soothing, sedative, and harmless tranquilizing effects, chamomile tea is a general toner for the uterus and helps relieve a number of gynecological complaints. When it comes to treating fibroids, chamomile is most useful for its ability to soothe frazzled nerves and promote a state of mind that is more conductive to healing.

Dose: Drink the tea freely (using one teaspoon of dried leaves per cup of water), and follow the dose instructions on capsule and tincture bottles.

Safety issues: None, unless you are using homeopathic substances. Wait two to three hours after taking the homeopathic remedy before using chamomile in any form.

Cramp bark (Viburnum opulus)

Cramp bark is a powerful antispasmodic, making it a great herb for regulating and relaxing the ovaries and uterus, thereby easing uterine pains and cramps. Some natural health-care practitioners recommend cramp bark in tea form during pregnancy for its possible ability to prevent miscarriage. Cramp bark is also thought to reduce blood loss during heavy periods.

Dose: The usual dose is two to three cups of the hot tea a day to relieve cramps. In fact, half a cup of the strong tea will relieve cramps, sometimes in as brief a period as twenty minutes. If you use the fluid extract, take ten to twenty drops, three times a day.

Safety issues: None.

Dong quai (Angelica sinensis)

An excellent tonic for maintaining and restoring gynecological health, this Chinese herb is also called "the female ginseng," because it nourishes and supports the ovaries, and helps balance hormone production throughout a woman's life. It also provides a good supply of iron, which is lost during heavy bleeding. Dong quai has been used by Asian healers for many centuries to cure many different female disorders, but it is most commonly prescribed to relieve premenstrual symptoms, menopausal symptoms, and painful menstrual cramping. Dong quai is also thought to act as an estrogen, and it does have some estrogenic effects. But we really do not know exactly how it works, because it does not seem to elevate estrogen levels. Dong quai should not be used by itself. In traditional Chinese medicine, it is always found in compounded tonics, along with other supporting herbs. Some compound formulas combine dong quai with chasteberry to balance hormone levels. Rehmannia and bupleurum are two commonly used Chinese herbs that are also often compounded with dong quai.

Dose: Dong quai is used in combination with other herbs in traditional Chinese botanical medicines, and does not cause problems in this form.

Safety issues: Though it is generally considered safe, some of dong quai's chemical components can interact with sunlight and cause a rash or severe sunburn. Women with fibroids who are experiencing heavy bleeding should avoid dong quai, as it could increase the blood flow. Dong quai is not recommended for pregnant or nursing women.

Echinacea (Echinacea angustifolia, purpurea, pallida)

This popular extract from the purple coneflower, a daisylike plant common to the American plains, is a known immune system toner and lymph system stimulant. This is why echinacea has come into the spotlight in the past several years, as increasing numbers of people complain of chronic fatigue and a variety of immunodeficiency diseases. I use echinacea in conjunction with other toning herbs to help remove toxins from the body and to improve general health, immunity, lymphatic flow, and energy. Once fibroid tumors are dissolving, echinacea compounds help the body rid itself of their toxic breakdown products. Some evidence even indicates that echinacea can help shrink fibroids.

Dose: Echinacea comes in a wide variety of forms. Some homeopathic doctors even prescribe injections of homeopathic echinacea formulations. Usually it is taken in fluid extract form, less often in capsule form. The usual dose for the extract is thirty drops, or one-half to one teaspoon, three times a day. If you take the capsules, I recommend 300 mg, three times a day.

Safety issues: None. The latest studies state that echinacea is safe when taken on a long-term basis. If you are healthy and your immune system is operating well, you do not need it. If your immune system is impaired, as evidenced by an infection, you can feel confident in taking this herb for as long as needed. Recent studies show that this herb is safe during pregnancy. Other studies suggest that if the immune system is impaired by such diseases as HIV, systemic lupus erythematosus, multiple sclerosis, and tuberculosis, echinacea could actually worsen these conditions by stimulating an already overstimulated system. Until more studies are done, avoid using echinacea if you suffer from these diseases.

Evening Primrose Oil (EPO) (Primula vulgaris)

Evening primrose is a rich and easily available source of linoleic acid and gamma-linolenic acid (GLA). Both are crucial to optimum gynecological function and hormone balance. As you may recall, your body also uses these essential fatty acids to make the hormones called prostaglandins (PGE 1) that regulate a wide range of body functions, including blood pressure, blood vessel tone, and cholesterol levels. Prostaglandins also reduce inflammation, maintain breast health, and diminish uterine cramping.

Evening primrose oil is recommended mainly to promote peak hormonal balance. If your levels of PGE 1 are low, you are liable to suffer from PMS, menstrual cramps, fibroids, and other gynecological conditions.

Initial experiments suggested that evening primrose oil is effective only when administered by injection. But recent research suggests that enteric-coated tablets are also effective, because that form enables the evening primrose to bypass the intestinal tract and deliver its ingredients directly to the bloodstream. Some researchers also consider evening primrose oil to be a good preventative and cure for cysts in the breasts and ovaries.

Dose: Take 1,000 to 3,000 mg evening primrose oil per day to provide about 250 mg of GLA. Some researchers have used as much as 6,000 mg per day, without any adverse effects. When combined with vitamin B_6 and vitamin E, evening primrose oil becomes a powerful weapon against PMS, which is often experienced by women with fibroid tumors. Take evening primrose oil with 50 mg of B_6 once a day, along with 400 to 800 IU of vitamin E a day, split into two or three doses. Magnesium, vitamin C, and zinc are also necessary for EPO to be effective.

Safety issues: High doses (as in 2,500 mg, three times a day) for too long a period (more than six to eight months) can offset the balance of your other prostaglandins. This can create more inflammatory, "bad" prostaglandins that could actually give you the opposite effect: hormonal imbalance and inflammation. If you are unsure about which fats you need to take, have your health-care practitioner do a red blood cell fatty acid analysis, to be analyzed by Great Smokies Diagnostic Laboratory in North Carolina.

Fenugreek (Trigonella foenumgraecum)

These tasty, nutritious seeds are found in various East Indian, Pakastani, and African dishes. But fenugreek was first prized by the ancient peoples of Asia and those living on the shores of the Mediterranean, because it is a valuable female tonic, blood sugar regulator, and antipollutant for the body. These seeds actually contain phytohormones, the hormonelike plant substances that help prevent the estrogen-dominant state that leads to fibroids and helps them to grow. Fenugreek also helps the pelvis discharge the excess mucus and the toxins trapped in it—a condition often associated with fibroids. Some herbalists even allege that it can be used in conjunction with other herbs to increase breast size without surgery. Turkish women still snack on a mixture of powdered fenugreek seeds and honey to maintain the gynecological health and fertility that fibroids can impede.

Dose: Fenugreek seed can be brewed into a tea that is a wonderful natural medicine for an impressive array of ailments. Steep two teaspoons of the seeds in a cup of boiling water for five minutes. Strain and add honey and/or lemon or lime juice. Drink freely. Use twenty to thirty drops, two to three times per day, of the tincture.

Safety issues: None, other than an upset stomach if more than 100 gm a day is taken.

Garlic (Allium sativum)

Whole garlic contains allicin, the sulphur-containing compound that gives garlic most of its beneficial properties. It is also rich in vitamins essential for optimum health: vitamin A, thiamine, riboflavin, and niacin. A close relative of the onion, garlic has a long and impressive history of service to human health, including gynecological health. Among its many wonderful benefits are regulating blood pressure, aiding circulation, detoxifying, lowering triglycerides, and relieving PMS, including PMS associated with fibroids. As an antiangiogenesis agent, garlic prevents tumors from growing new blood vessels, which also makes it a cancer preventer. Garlic has been shown to reduce the incidence of several gastrointestinal cancers.

Garlic also helps stop the growth of fibroids. Fibroids and other foreign growths in the body support themselves by increasing blood flow in order to bring in more nutrients and help eliminate waste. Garlic is the agent that thwarts that plan. This pungent bulb can also relieve painful menstruation, most likely by its ability to reduce platelet adhesion and keep blood more fluid.

Dose: Commercial garlic preparations should contain a daily dose of at least 5,000 mcg of allicin, garlic's active medicinal ingredient. You can also eat this pungent bulb freely, with the ideal amount being about one clove a day. Use it as a seasoning for your food.

Most brands of garlic capsules, tablets, and liquids are specially processed to be odorless.

Safety issues: Too much garlic can irritate the intestinal tract, and studies using rats found that very large amounts of garlic over very long periods of time caused anemia, weight loss, and failure to grow. Garlic also has a blood-thinning effect, so it should be used with caution if you are taking any other blood-thinning pharmaceutical drugs, such as aspirin or Coumadin, or blood-thinning natural supplements, such as ginkgo biloba or fish oils, unless under the supervision of a health-care practitioner. Garlic is not contraindicated during pregnancy and nursing. In fact, it seems that breast-feeding is more effective when nursing mothers include garlic in their diets.

Ginger (Zingiber officinale)

Ginger is native to southern Asia and has been used in China for medicinal purposes for thousands of years. It is served along with the hot green mustard called wasabi, whenever you eat sushi made with raw fish, in order to prevent parasitic disease. Hot ginger poultices are used by traditional Asian healers to relieve congestion anywhere in the body. I have used these poultices on the outer part of the vagina during childbirth to prevent tears and to speed postdelivery healing. Gingerroot is classified as a stimulant that jumpstarts the endocrine glands that are key to maintaining optimum hormone balance. It is also a useful anti-inflammatory and is wonderfully effective against nausea and motion sickness. Recent studies confirm that ginger lowers cholesterol levels even more effectively than onion or garlic. As an anti-inflammatory and modulator of prostaglandins, ginger can help discourage "bad" prostaglandins and reduce the severe menstrual cramps that can accompany fibroid conditions. Ginger tea is also a delicious and energizing replacement for coffee.

Dose: Gingerroot can be grated and used as a condiment or brewed as a tea that can be drunk freely. Experiment to see how much relieves your nausea, indigestion, or circulation problems. Usual doses are 2 to 4 gm a day. The fresh root is probably the most effective, but if the whole root is not available at your local health food store or Asian grocery, you can find ginger in capsules and tinctures. Follow dose instructions on the bottle label. Ginger is also used in compound herbal formulas to enhance effectiveness.

Safety issues: If large amounts are taken on an empty stomach, ginger can irritate the gastrointestinal tract. Studies have found that taking as much as 6 gm of dried powdered root at a time, over prolonged periods, can damage the intestinal lining and possibly lead to ulcers. Doses as high as 10 gm per day have been shown to interfere with platelet aggregation and could cause a blood-clotting problem if you are about to undergo surgery. Since ginger heats the body, it also should not be used if you are suffering from hot flashes.

Ginseng root, Panax (Panax quinquefolius or Panax schinseng)

This venerable herb is a true toner and energizer that restores overall strength, muscle tone, and vitality in those who are chronically fatigued or have been weakened by illness, including the excessive bleeding and cramping associated with fibroid conditions. Ginseng proponents make numerous claims for its healing and strengthening abilities, including its ability to maintain optimum and steady blood pressure, blood sugar, metabolism, and energy levels. The active ginsenosides stimulate the immune system. Ginseng has enjoyed a centuries-old reputation in Asia and the Americas as an aphrodisiac because it directly benefits gynecological function. Panax ginseng is naturally found in both Asia and North America. The beauty of panax ginseng is that it supports the adrenal glands and aids toleration of stress, which is why it is classified as an adaptogen. Most adaptogen herbs can be taken for as long as you like. However, I do not recommend panax ginseng for women who are already overstimulated and anxious, as this herb can actually increase anxiety in those overstimulated women.

Dose: Ginseng is best taken in the morning because of its stimulating action. Various roots differ widely in their effectiveness. Generally, the more expensive the root, the more effectively it works and the lower the risk of irritation. You can chew the root, drink the tea, take the powder or mix it in your food, sip an extract, or swallow capsules.

Dose depends on the content of ginsenoside, the active ingredient in panax ginseng. Select a brand that is standardized to give you at least 5 percent of ginsenosides. Ginsana is one of the best formulations of ginseng available, but many others also work well. Take one capsule a day to maintain ginsenoside levels in your bloodstream. One dose of the standardized extract—ten to fifteen drops—will do the same.

Safety issues: Ginseng has the advantage of being perfectly safe over long-term use. But if you suffer from high blood pressure, your pressure could rise when you take this root. Women taking panax ginseng may experience breast tenderness. Reduce the dose and the pain will vanish. Be aware that if you use this herb along with other stimulants, such as caffeine, you can become overstimulated. Long-term use in some women can cause menstrual abnormalities. I do not recommend that pregnant or nursing women use ginseng.

Ginseng, Siberian (Eleutherococcus senticosus)

Siberian ginseng is actually an entirely different herb from panax ginseng. Yet it is also a good energizer and stress reliever (whether that stress has physical or emotional causes). Siberian ginseng also tones the adrenals, thereby strengthening gynecological function and promoting hormone balance. It is also well suited for long-term use.

Dose: Drink ginseng tea, chew the root, take capsules or tablets, ingest the extract, or mix it into various beverages. A recent study found that the extract and powder forms are more effective than fresh-sliced ginseng, its juice, or tea, particularly if that extract is made from high-grade roots. Take two capsules, twice a day, or thirty drops of the fluid extract a day. Some health experts suggest taking Siberian ginseng for six to eight weeks, then stopping for one to two weeks before taking it again. I have put patients on this herb for six months straight, without any negative effects.

Safety issues: Large amounts of this herb can lead to loose stools, and, if it is taken too close to bedtime, it can cause insomnia. But Siberian ginseng is a very safe herb that can even be used by pregnant and nursing women. Be aware that this is not the case for Siberian ginseng's soundalike—but very different—cousin, panax ginseng, which should not be used during pregnancy or while nursing.

Licorice root (Glycyrrhiza glabra)

Known as "the great harmonizer" in Chinese medicine, this tasty root sweetens many tonic formulas. It is also a great anti-inflammatory, toner, and energizer for the entire body, particularly for the adrenal glands, mainly by virtue of its most active medicinal ingredient, glycyrrhizin, which has a similar structural appearance to adrenal cortical hormones. Licorice root also normalizes estrogen metabolism, inhibiting estrogen action when estrogens are too high and boosting its action when estrogen levels are too low. Therefore, it is a good aid for preventing and halting the growth of fibroids. It also has antiallergic and anti-inflammatory properties.

Many health-minded ex-smokers chew on this root to calm their tobacco cravings, at the same time that they are toning their organs and promoting better gum health. Some traditional cultures use licorice root to increase fertility.

Dose: Licorice root is available in whole form in health food stores and Asian herbal stores. It is also widely available in tea, capsule, and tincture form. The dose is based on the content level of its active ingredients, particularly glycyrrhizin, and also on your blood pressure. Licorice can increase blood pressure, so you need to monitor your intake in order to find the amount that works for you. Standard dose is one to three capsules, two to three times a day.

Safety issues: Licorice root can increase blood pressure and cause water retention. Do not take it if you have hypertension, a history of renal failure, or use digitalis preparations. Another form of licorice root called deglycyrrhizinated licorice (DGL), can be used even if you have high blood pressure. This form is also used instead of antacids to relieve gastritis, or inflammation of the stomach, and reflux esophagitis.

Red raspberry (Rubus idaeus)

This is one of my favorite herbs for many women's gynecological problems. Many holistic health practitioners use it successfully during pregnancy. It is also helpful in treating gynecological problems, especially fibroids and abnormal uterine bleeding, because raspberry strengthens and tones the uterus. Red raspberry is an all-around great herb for female problems of almost every kind, because of its soothing action and its astringent properties, due to its high content of plant tannins. This makes it especially useful for women with fibroids because it will help reduce heavy menstrual flow and ease uterine cramps. These same astringent properties also make red raspberry leaves a good choice for treating diarrhea. The tea is said to help prevent miscarriage and relieve morning sickness.

Dose: Red raspberry is available in bulk, tea bags, and, for healing purposes, in capsule and tincture forms. The usual dose for the tea is three cups a day. In tincture form, take one teaspoon up to three times a day.

Safety issues: Red raspberry is a very safe herb that can be used without fear of negative effects.

Red clover (Trifolium pratense)

Red clover has been in the natural healer's medicine bag since the Greeks and Romans. Like soy, red clover's active ingredients include natural plant hormones like genistein that compete for hormone receptor sites against stronger, potentially more harmful estrogens. This makes red clover especially effective in healing and preventing fibroid tumors, as well as other conditions related to estrogen dominance. Studies continue to suggest that the isoflavones genistein, daidzein, and coumestans also inhibit cancer formation and help reduce the incidence of hormone-dependent cancers. They also interfere with estrogens' growth-enhancing effects on uterine and fibroid tissue.

Dose: Take one cup of the tea, three times a day, or one-half to one teaspoon of the fluid extract, three times a day. Take one to two capsules of the herb, two times per day. Promensil, a commercial red clover preparation often used for menopause support, supplies 40 mg of isoflavones and is taken once a day.

Safety issues: Red clover is relatively safe, but very high doses in animals can interfere with fertility. In one study, sheep that grazed only on red clover did have reproductive problems. However, this dose was way in excess of any amount women would use.

Sarsaparilla (Smilax officinalis)

Clinical reports indicate that sarsaparilla root and berries tone the reproductive organs and glands and increase sex drive and energy, possibly because of the herb's progesteronelike effect. Sarsaparilla is an excellent tonic herb that can be taken for weeks or months in order to restore strength and vitality. Because it also supports progesterone levels, it is also an effective hormone balancer.

Dose: Take this herb in tea form, capsule, or extract as a general daily tonic, for months at a time. The usual dose is ten drops of extract in the morning and evening, after meals. Or take one capsule in the morning and one in the evening, after meals. You can also drink three cups of tea a day.

Safety issues: In rare instances, sarsaparilla can cause stomach irritation. Sarsaparilla can also interfere with the absorption and/or elimination of drugs like digitialis and bismuth, so care should be taken if you are using these drugs.

Saw palmetto (Serenoa repens)

Saw palmetto is a small palm tree native to the West Indies and the Atlantic coast of North America from South Carolina to Florida. Native Americans used saw palmetto berries to treat genitourinary tract disturbances and, as a tonic, to nutritionally support the entire body. More recently, it has been touted as a male herb to help reduce benign swelling and inflammation of the prostate gland, but saw palmetto is also effective for maintaining women's hormone balance, which makes it helpful in healing fibroids. Women have also used it to correct disorders of the mammary glands, and traditional healers claim that long-term use causes the breasts to enlarge, decreases uterine cramps, and restores tone to the uterus. Actually, this herb is helpful for treating virtually all diseases of the reproductive system. I have used saw palmetto in combination with other herbs to treat polycystic ovary disease, especially when there is evidence of male hormone effect, such as excessive hair growth.

Dose: Take one 80 to 200 mg capsule after each meal. Make sure the capsule is standardized to give 85 percent to 95 percent of fatty acid sterols. The key to getting enough saw palmetto is the standardization from a reputable brand. Some herbalists believe you must take the whole berry.

Safety issues: None, although, as is the case with many other nontoxic herbs, a large amount of saw palmetto taken on an empty stomach, over a long period of time, can cause stomach irritation.

Squaw vine (Mitchella repens)

I have used squaw vine (also known as partridgeberry) in combination with red raspberry, which is known for its astringent properties, in cases of heavy vaginal bleeding. It also seems to relieve cramping associated with menstrual periods and reduce pelvic congestion. These properties make squaw vine a helpful herb for treating fibroids. It can also be effective in cases of infertility related to hormone imbalance.

Dose: As a tea, squaw vine can be taken three times a day. Or take thirty drops of the tincture, two to three times a day.

Safety issues: None.

Valerian root (Valeriana officinalis)

This is one of my favorite herbs for insomnia, but some people think it smells like old gym socks. The Alvita preparation takes care of that problem by combining valerian with mint for a great bedtime brew. Valerian root has been used throughout Western history to treat everything from stomach discomfort to migraines to the plague. Its primary effect, though, is sedative because it relaxes muscles and nerves. Some herbalists recommend stuffing your pillow with this root to promote a peaceful night's sleep and the relaxed state of mind that is most conducive to healing fibroids. Although the names are similar, valerian root is not related to the tranquilizer Valium.

Dose: Valerian root can be taken as a tea, capsule, or tincture. The usual dose is two capsules, one cup of the tea, or ten to fifteen drops of the tincture, taken half an hour before bedtime. Another option is to take a long, warm bath infused with fifteen to twenty drops of valerian decoction or oil.

Safety issues: Valerian is approved by the United States Food and Drug Administration because studies show that it does not impair driving ability or lead to addiction. It is also fine during pregnancy from the second trimester on.

TRADITIONAL COMPOUND TONIC REMEDIES

Compound tonic remedies mix a group of herbs together so that their synergistic effect balances and stimulates particular body systems. Because they are used together, the chance of negative effects from any single herb is likely to be countered by the positive action of another. Tonics make wonderful preventative treatments that also enhance vitality and well-being. But they are equally effective even after disease or dysfunction, including fibroid tumors, has already set in.

If you are susceptible to gynecological weakness in the sex organs and glands or are over forty, it is a good idea to make an herbal tonic formula part of your daily routine. It usually takes a few weeks to bring any body system into balance, and the effects should last for several months.

Tonics can also be a good idea before forty. Modern women often combine the demands of full-time careers with the stresses of full-time family care. They would be wise to take tonics for at least two

weeks out of every month to promote strength, energy, healthy adrenal glands, liver detoxification, a hardy nervous system, and hormone balance. Do not take a tonic formula during pregnancy,
unless under the supervision of a health-care practitioner.

Essiac is a compound tonic that draws on the healing wisdom of
an Ojibwa Indian shaman and contains traditional North American
herbs that are still popular today—burdock, slippery elm, sheep
sorrel, and turkey rhubarb. This tonic was named after the Cana-
dian nurse named Rene Caisse (Essiac is her name spelled backward) who witnessed an Indian healer in Canada use it to heal a
woman with breast cancer. Caisse then brought the tonic to the
States. Essiac is too complex to make on your own, but it is available
at some health food stores and through mail order companies. Flor-
essence is another compound tonic that is similar to Essiac.

HOMEMADE TONIC RECIPES

The following are easy-to-make tonics you can make yourself to
enhance your gynecological health. Any one of them can easily become part of your regular diet.

Chinese chicken soup

For this simple recipe, you need whole, fresh dong quai, which
can be purchased in Chinese markets and herb stores. Place one to
two heads of the herb (about one inch in size) in chicken broth or
soup, and season as desired. Simmer in a slow cooker for approximately three to five hours.

Fennel-licorice hormone tonic

Simmer two teaspoons of slightly crushed fennel seeds and one
ounce of minced licorice root in one pint of water for twenty minutes. Let stand until cool. Strain. Take two tablespoons, twice a day.

Hops-citrus hormone tonic

Simmer the peels of two lemons and one orange in one quart of
water for twenty minutes. Add three tablespoons of dried hops and

simmer for three minutes. Remove from heat and stir in honey to taste. Cover and cool to lukewarm. Add three tablespoons of lecithin, mixing well. Take half a cup, three or four times a day. (This tonic will increase breast milk flow in nursing mothers.)

American Indian tonic gruel

Bring two tablespoons of unrefined oatmeal (which tonifies the uterus and ovaries), half a cup of raisins, and one quart of water to a boil. Cover and simmer for forty-five minutes. Remove from heat and strain. Add honey to taste. Cool and add half a teaspoon of lemon juice.

Fenugreek seed with honey tonic treats

This valuable seed is rich in vitamin A, which helps regulate menstrual flow and heal the body's mucous membranes. Since these seeds also contain a chemical that acts like a hormone in frogs and speeds up flower production in plants, many cultures also believe that fenugreek regulates human female hormone levels. You can brew the tea (see page 154) or try these tasty honey treats.

Grind the seeds into a powder. (Use a coffee grinder or a blender at high speed, or try an old-fashioned mortar and pestle.) Mix with an equal part of honey.

Sesame combination tonic treat

This delicious dessert paste is a quick energy tonic and hormone booster. Simmer three tablespoons of sesame seed, one ounce of licorice root, and one-quarter pound of pitted, minced dates in two quarts of water until the liquid is reduced to one quart. Remove from heat and add one cup of honey, stirring well until the mixture is well blended.

Dose: Take two tablespoons three or four times a day, or as needed.

Safety issues: None.

Fibroid-Healing Herbs

We have talked about tonic herbs and compounded herbs, many of which are extremely helpful in treating fibroid conditions. Some herbs work directly on the uterus, ovaries, and even on the fibroids themselves. Other herbs help heal fibroid conditions by boosting adrenal gland function, which encourages proper hormone balance. Other herbs are useful because they enhance liver function, especially by helping the liver metabolize and remove toxins that bind to estrogen receptor sites in the uterus and fibroids. Still other herbal remedies tone the immune and lymphatic systems to help the body regularly eliminate waste products built up by the fibroids. Again, the body behaves as if each part was connected by a web of interaction. This is important to keep in mind, because any weakness in only one part of that web will inevitably affect the others. For example, if you eat well, exercise regularly, think positive thoughts, but have only three bowel movements a week, waste will still—literally—back up.

ADRENAL GLAND BOOSTERS

Siberian ginseng, nettles, licorice, and wild yam all boost adrenal gland function, thereby helping your body maintain the peak hormone balance that prevents fibroids and halts their growth. These herbs also help women cope with the stress of a fibroid condition. You can drink them as teas if your adrenals are not overly weak. Tinctures (fluid extracts) are better if your adrenals are severely weakened by stress and/or illness. Take two or three cups of the tea, or thirty drops of the tincture, two to three times a day, or two capsules, twice a day. (You will learn even more ways to strengthen your adrenal glands in a later chapter.)

LIVER DETOXIFIERS AND STRENGTHENERS

Herbs most commonly used to nourish and tone the liver include dandelion root, yellow dock, burdock root, and milk thistle. Artichoke is another excellent herb that supports the liver, and it also helps reduce cholesterol levels. These herbs prevent fatty buildup in the liver that can interfere with its detoxification functions. Silymarin, the active principle in milk thistle, is a major antioxidant for the liver. It also helps the production of glutathione, an antioxidant that supports healthy estrogen metabolism. The other herbs act as blood cleaners and, by preventing fatty buildup in the liver, they also support healthy gallbladder function. All these actions support healthy waste removal and hormone balance. The tonics can be taken as teas, capsules, or tinctures, depending on the severity of your condition.

FIBROID SHRINKERS

Chasteberry (vitex) and the Grifron company's maitake mushroom D fraction are both reported to shrink small subserous (surface) and intramural fibroids. Studies show that the maitake mushroom D fraction inhibits the growth of cells, including fibroid cells. It even has been used successfully in cancer therapy. Vitex is a wonderful tonic for the entire reproductive system that works at the level of the pituitary gland. It increases LH production, which helps increase the body's levels of progesterone. As you already know, progesterone levels must be high enough to balance estrogen, in order to avoid an estrogen-dominant state that can lead to fibroids. Studies show that vitex can reduce the size of small fibroids, but it is less effective on larger fibroid tumors. This is just one compelling reason for treating fibroids while they are still small, before they grow into a serious health threat.

Fibroid-healing compound formulas like Scudder's Alternative, Echinacea/Red Root formula, and Fraxinus (also known as white ash), in combination with red root (also known as ceanothus), are also helpful in halting fibroid growth. They are all available through Gaia Herbs. (See the appendix.) These formulas work by combining several different herbs that tone the lymphatic system. They help remove toxins from the body, support liver function, enhance cell metabolism, lower cell growth, and reduce pelvic congestion.

All of these benefits combine to help shrink fibroids. Another compounded herbal remedy that has become more difficult to obtain is
Turska's Formula. It combines four herbs: aconite, bryonia, phytolacca, and gelsemium. Bryonia has become an endangered species,
but you get a combination of gelsemium and phytolacca (*aka* poke
weed), which has also been shown to reduce the size of fibroids.
Gaia Herbs recently produced a bryonia product without endanger-
ing that herb's presence in the wild. Their gelsemium/phytolacca
compound also contains bryonia and aconite. However, these herbs
have been shown to be potentially toxic, so take no more than five
drops, two to three times a day, and only under the watchful eye of
a knowledgeable health-care practitioner. In any case, you cannot
get these herbs except by prescription from a medical doctor (M.D.)
or naturopathic physician (N.D.). The Scudder's Formula, echi-
nacea/red root, and fraxinus/ceanothus are nontoxic compound
remedies that can be used at a dose of thirty drops, two to three
times a day, without any negative effects.

Make sure you occasionally interrupt courses of the above
herbs, having short breaks without them. This way you allow your
body to continue receiving the herbs' full benefits, without the risk
of developing a sensitivity. Take the herbs for a few months at a
time, and then stop for one to two weeks. Some herbs should be
taken separately, but the herbs described above work well in combination.

UTERINE DECONGESTANTS

Other herbs heal fibroids by helping to remove toxins from a
congested uterus so it can function more efficiently and be less
prone to fibroids and other tumors. These herbs include partridgeberry (*Mitchella repens*), false unicorn root (*helonias*), and prickly
ash, which is included in many compound formulas to increase
blood and lymph circulation so toxins can be efficiently eliminated
from the pelvis. The major reason why many women with fibroids
undergo surgery is excessive bleeding.

Many women consult me for hormone replacement therapy after they have already undergone a hysterectomy because their fibroids would not stop bleeding. Yet I have found, in most cases, that bleeding due to fibroids can be controlled through some of the wonderful herbs nature has given us. My favorite astringent, or blood-controlling, herbs include red raspberry, yarrow, and shepherd's purse, also known as capsella. Other astringent herbs—lady's mantle (alchemilla), cranesbill (geranium), and cinnamon—work nearly as well. I tell women with heavy bleeding associated with fibroids to take thirty drops each of yarrow and red raspberry tinctures, two to three times a day, for about two weeks prior to the expected onset of menstruation. When their period starts, they continue with the herbs. If the bleeding is still excessive, they can add the same amount of shepherd's purse.

One woman bled so heavily that she had to keep jumping in the shower to wash away the blood that was coursing down her legs. After three to four doses of the three herbs I just described, the bleeding stopped suddenly. If you need a remedy immediately and cannot get these herbs, use cinnamon, which also does well as an astringent herb. Mix two to three teaspoons in a cup of hot water. Drink, and repeat every thirty minutes, until the bleeding slows.

Some of these herbs may not be familiar to you, but most of them can be found at your local health food and/or herb stores or through mail order and Internet Web site catalogs. (See the resource guide.) Again, I cannot stress enough the importance of avoiding mass-market brands like GNC, Costco, and Price Club.

Although I am not a homeopath, several homeopathic remedies are also helpful in reducing the excessive bleeding that accompanies fibroid conditions. I have used sepia, sabina, nux vomica, phosphorus, and that old standby belladona with success. The standard strength is 30C. Homeopathic remedies are designed to work in very specific situations, so it is best to consult a homeopath who can find the right remedy for you.

7

Fibroid-Healing Exercises and Bodywork

It was not too long ago that women were discouraged from exercising because they would develop "masculine" musculature. Today, we recognize that exercise is essential to good health. Our concept of exercise is also expanding, as interest builds in such traditional eastern body-mind disciplines as yoga, chi gong, and tai chi and other martial arts. Still, we are just beginning to understand the equation between exercise and health and exploring the possibility that certain specific exercises can be of special benefit to the healing of gynecological conditions like fibroids.

This chapter will describe the exercises that are most supportive of gynecological health in simple, easy-to-follow terms. Most of these exercises help heal fibroids by promoting overall health, lymphatic and blood circulation, and hormonal balance. But the healing benefits of exercise are really limitless.

✦ Betty's Story

Betty was a thirty-eight-year-old stay-at-home mom with three young children. Her last pregnancy and delivery had been especially difficult, and, two years later, she was still carrying forty extra pounds. Betty's self-image was at an all-time low. She was overweight, her husband was not interested in making love, and her post-delivery belly was so large that she still looked pregnant.

Until her annual checkup with her gynecologist, Betty did not know that her huge belly was due, at least in part, to a sixteen-weeks-size multifibroid uterine condition. Those fibroids were also the reason why heavy bleeding, pain, and bloating were making her monthly periods a nightmare.

The size of Betty's fibroids meant her situation qualified as an emergency, but I thought that a total fibroid-healing program might save her from surgery. I recommended several lifestyle changes, including a hormone-balancing diet, supplements, herbs, natural hormones, and regular exercise.

"I haven't got time for exercise," Betty objected at first. I was able to persuade her to join a gym. Because baby-sitting was a problem, she could attend only one class a week. The solution was exercise videotapes to use at home and regular walks with her husband and children.

After a few months, Betty's condition improved enough to save her from surgery. She had lost weight, her belly had reduced considerably, her self-esteem was better, and her menstrual symptoms were much less troublesome. A total healing plan had helped to shrink Betty's fibroid uterus down to the more manageable size of a fourteen-weeks pregnancy. If she kept to her program, there was every reason to expect her fibroids to shrink even more.

Let us take a look at the role exercise played in Betty's success story, and why it is such an important component of fibroid healing.

How Exercise Helps You Heal Fibroids

• *Improved circulation and elimination.* All exercise boosts the body's circulatory and elimination systems and oxygenates the system down to the cellular level. This is where essential life functions are performed, including the formation of healthy hormone-receptor-site complexes.

• *Reduced risk for chronic illness.* Exercise helps virtually every body part perform better. It reduces the risk for so many chronic conditions that if exercise were a pill, it would be the most prescribed medicine in this country.

• *Reduced stress.* When exercise is done correctly, it is a great stress reducer. Poorly managed stress has been proven in scientific studies to set off hormonal chain reactions that can lead to hormone-imbalance-related conditions like fibroids. Common stress factors include physical illness, hypoglycemia, job and career worries, financial pressures, relationship problems, the death of a loved one, and other life-altering events, such as a major move or your upcoming wedding.

Believe it or not, though, too much exercise can impair your health. In our society, if a moderate amount of something is deemed beneficial, we tend to go overboard with it, reasoning that a lot of this something must be even better. I have seen women exercise to excess and create for themselves such problems as severe osteoporosis, chronic fatigue, general impaired health, and hormonal imbalance. Nevertheless, regular, moderate exercise is one of the best ways to discharge stress.

• *Improved hormone production.* Regular exercise improves hormone production. Some experts theorize that regular exercisers may experience an increase in the adrenal hormone DHEA, which is linked to better energy levels and hormone balance. When we are under constant stress, our adrenal glands are continually releasing stress hormones. They also have to work overtime to keep up other hormone production. The major hormone released when we are under stress is cortisol. Progesterone is a precursor hormone for the production of cortisol. If the body needs a lot of cortisol to cope with constant stress, too much of the adrenal glands' production of progesterone will be used to make cortisol. Not enough progesterone will be left to counter the effects of estrogen in the body. This is one of the reasons chronic stress inevitably leads to the estrogen-dominant state that allows fibroids to develop and grow.

• *Diminished effects of hormone imbalance.* Regular, moderate exercise—both strengthening and flexibility-promoting types—helps regulate menstrual periods and reduce the various symptoms of the conditions that can result from an estrogen-dominant state, including fibroids.

• *More endorphins.* Researchers note that immediately after a workout, blood levels of endorphins rise considerably. Endorphins are the body's feel-good hormones, natural painkillers that also promote a feeling of well-being that helps counter fibroid-related cramps, pain, and depression. Anyone who has experienced "runner's high" knows that exercise reduces anxiety and banishes mild depression. You do not have to run several miles a day or perform difficult aerobics moves. A brisk walk for twenty to thirty minutes in natural surroundings is enough to raise the body's endorphin levels and reduce fibroid-related tension and cramping via the same mechanism as runner's high.

• *Better overall muscle tone.* Better muscle tone helps prevent your body from locking into painful cramps, a common symptom suffered by women with serious fibroid conditions.

• *Greater flexibility.* Yoga, stretch routines, and other flexibility exercises are also especially helpful for reducing cramping associated with fibroids.

• *Improved self-image.* We all want to be loved for our inner selves, and we should be. But there is nothing wrong with a modest dose of "healthy" vanity. Keeping your body strong and fit boosts your self-image, thus motivating you to take even better care of your body and regard it as your temple.

• *Regular bowel movements.* Regular exercise helps keep us regular, so that hormones the liver "packages" for excretion are eliminated safely and regularly. This helps maintain hormone balance.

Types of Exercise

Aerobic exercise—running, walking, swimming, or biking—specifically boosts cardiovascular and respiratory functions. "Aerobic" means that the body and muscles consume oxygen while the exercise is being performed. This aids the body's efforts to process and use sugars and carbohydrates for fuel. By helping the body use sugars and carbs more efficiently, aerobic exercise also helps normalize insulin levels and prevent hormonal imbalance caused by high insulin levels. Whenever you do aerobic exercise, evaluate your pulse before, during, and after your workout. The easiest place to feel your pulse is on the inside of your wrist, with the palm of the hand facing up. Place the tips of the index and middle fingers of your left hand in a line along the thumb side of the right wrist, starting about one inch from the crease between the palm and wrist. Push down firmly with those two fingers so you can feel the pulsation without muffling it. The pulse rate you should aim for during exercise is calculated by subtracting your age from 220, then multiplying the result by .6 to .8. Beginners should multiply by .6; more advanced exercisers can multiply by .7 or .8.

Aerobic exercise also enhances gynecological health by facilitating your body's natural cleansing systems, oxygen delivery, and hormone production.

Weight training improves muscular health, reverses osteoporosis, and strengthens the muscles that support the uterus. Weight training is an anaerobic exercise, which means that it does not utilize oxygen while you are performing it. This type of exercise aids the body's ability to utilize fats for fuel. This latter benefit is the reason anaerobic or weight-bearing exercise becomes so important during the perimenopause and menopausal years, when maintaining a healthy weight is an important issue.

Yoga, tai chi, chi gong, and other traditional Eastern disciplines stretch, tone, and oxygenate the body's organs and glands. They also are designed to dramatically increase the flow of energy, or "chi," to the pelvic organs and hormone glands. Chi, in the Chinese tradition, refers to life-force energy. This is the same energy the Japanese call ki, Hindus refer to as prana, Jews call chai, and Christians call Christ consciousness. Traditional Eastern healers and philosophers have understood for many centuries the profound connection between physical exercise and the flow of chi in the body. If chi flows freely because the body is exercised properly, the health of the pelvic organs and hormone levels will be optimal. Some of these exercises also act as effective pain relievers. At the same time, they strengthen and heal your pelvic organs and hormone glands.

Pilates is a relatively new exercise technique that seems to hold promise because it combines the health-enhancing benefits of strengthening and flexibility techniques.

Warning: Do not overdo it. Again, too much exercise or overly vigorous exercise can be health depleting by robbing you of stamina and energy you need for health and healing.

✦ Connie's Story

As I write the above warning, I am reminded of Connie, a New York City psychotherapist who came to see me when she was going through menopause. Connie stood about five feet tall and weighed a trim 97 pounds. After spending an entire day helping people sort out their emotional issues, she loved to run through Central Park and let off the stress. Rain or shine, Connie clocked five hard miles a day.

Connie's strict exercise regimen made her all the more perplexed about a recent bone density test result that showed she was losing bone mass. Despite good nutrition, adequate supplements, hormone replacement therapy, and regular exercise, Connie had osteoporosis. It took several months for me to convince Connie that her overly ambitious running program was the reason for this condition. Those five miles a day were actually working against her. Instead of helping her build up bone, the lengthy, strenuous runs were breaking down her bone and muscle tissues. After vigorous exercise, a certain amount of bone and muscle tissue always breaks down. The body needs time to recuperate and to make repairs. During that rest cycle, bone and tissue build up again and become even stronger than before, but Connie was not allowing her body enough time to effect this buildup. Instead, her daily exercise program was continually breaking down bone and muscle. Overexercising can also exhaust your body, creating additional health problems, including hormonal imbalance so severe that you can stop menstruating.

Western Exercises for a Stronger, More Flexible Torso

What society may consider the "perfect" body is not necessarily the healthiest body. We are not concerned here with ideal body proportions or with artificial body part enhancements that conform to fantasy media images of the sexy woman. Regular, moderate exercise improves overall health, stamina, and self-confidence. It helps you become stronger, more toned, and flexible, and it primes your body to heal.

Any good trainer at a gym can provide you with an effective workout program, but be sure to include the following exercises that have direct impact on gynecological health. Always remember to inhale and exhale evenly while performing any exercise. Exhale during the strenuous part of the exercise. If you do not blow out during the difficult phase of an exercise movement, you risk damaging your organs and creating more health problems. *Never hold your breath.*

PELVIC TILTS

This exercise strengthens your back, abdominal muscles, and buttocks.

- Lie on your back, bend your knees, and place your feet flat on the floor, shoulder-width apart.
- Squeeze your buttock muscles tightly, at the same time contracting your abdominal muscles and pressing the small of your back into the floor.

- Still pressing the small of your back into the floor, exhale as you push your hips up toward the ceiling. Continue pushing your hips upward, maintaining the contraction in your butt and abs, while keeping your upper back and feet on the floor. Hold at the highest point for a moment.
- Slowly lower to the floor, unrolling your spine from the middle down to the bottom, then lowering your buttocks.

Start out with five repetitions and gradually work your way up to twenty. Rest for thirty seconds, then repeat.

ABDOMINAL CRUNCHES

This exercise is an effective and safe way to tone and strengthen your abdominal muscles and lower back. Crunches also prevent and correct lower back pain and weakness often associated with gynecological weakness and fibroid conditions. They can also help repair the separation that sometimes develops in abdominal muscles after childbirth. This condition, known as *rectus diastasis*, appears almost as an indentation in the abdominal wall that runs vertically from the belly button to the pubic bone. Not only is it unattractive, it also contributes to poor abdominal muscle tone, and weakens the health of intra-abdominal organs.

- Lie on your back, knees bent and feet flat on the floor, in the same position as above.
- Contract your buttocks, at the same time pressing your lower back into the floor.
- Extend your arms along your sides. Exhale as you raise your upper body, at the same time contracting your abs and pressing your lower spine into the floor. Gently take hold of the upper part of each inner thigh.
- Keeping your body in the same raised position—lower spine pressed into the floor, abs contracted—bend your elbows and lightly touch your hands to your ears.

- Continue to press your lower spine against the floor and contract your abs for the count of six.
- Relax back down to the floor.

Work your way up to twenty crunches, twice a day. When you do these exercises the correct way, you should feel a "burn" sensation in your stomach muscles after you have finished. An easy way to augment your ab workout is with a "wheel" device that is used facing the floor, on your knees. Hold onto either side of the wheel device and roll it forward, all the way out, then use your abs to pull the wheel back in again. I am sure you have all seen variations of this simple device advertised in television infomercials. I recommend the wheel manufactured by Bollinger. It costs no more than a few dollars and works quite well. (See the appendix.)

BEST WESTERN EXERCISES FOR HEALTH

- Strength training: calisthenics, isometrics, weights, machines, Pilates, tae bo, and other martial arts.
- Aerobic activity: running, walking, cycling; aerobics classes; skiing and ski machines; jumping with a rope or mini-trampoline; swimming; and martial arts.
- Sports: dancing, skating, gymnastics; tennis and other racquet sports.

KEGEL EXERCISES

The pubococcygeus muscle, aka the PC muscle, located in the genital area between the vagina and the anal opening, should be strengthened and toned if you want to improve lifelong gynecological health. Traditional Eastern disciplines offer a myriad of exercises for this muscle, designed to increase tone in the pelvic organs, improve circulation, and balance hormone levels. The West has only one exercise: Kegels. But Kegel exercises are quite effective when practiced regularly. They tone pelvic muscles and bring increased amounts of blood into and out of the pelvis. This helps keep toxins and congestion in the pelvis at a minimum, thereby reducing the risk of fibroid development and helping to keep existing fibroids in check.

Kegeling, which was developed by the physician Arnold Kegel as a technique to correct incontinence, involves rhythmically contracting and relaxing the PC muscle, as if you were trying to stop the flow of urine.

THE BENEFITS OF KEGELING

Like any other muscle that is exercised regularly, the PC muscle will become healthier and more toned, and develop a richer blood and nerve supply. Not only will healthy blood flow throughout the pelvis increase nutrient intake and reduce congestion, the bladder will become stronger, which helps prevent embarrassing and dismaying loss of urine. All this translates into improved gynecological health and fibroid healing.

WHEN TO KEGEL

Another great thing about Kegeling is that the exercises can be done anywhere, anytime, in front of anyone, and no one will be the wiser.

Establishing a regular Kegeling routine is up to you. You can trick yourself into a daily routine by linking Kegel sessions to other daily activities. Here are some suggestions:

- While showering or in the bath. (If women combine Kegeling with a fifteen-minute soak in a saltwater bath—using one cup sea salt or Epsom salts to a full tub of warm water—they are also cultivating an ideal vaginal environment.)
- While brushing and flossing. (The advantage of linking these two chores is that most of us do not take enough time to

clean our teeth thoroughly. This helps you to do both beneficial activities longer. It is also a good exercise in coordination—like patting your head and rubbing your tummy at the same time.)

• Before or after every meal. Kegeling at these times could serve as a weight-loss tool and aid to digestion by reminding you not to rush through your meals.

• While waiting for a traffic light to change or waiting to pay a bridge or tunnel toll. Doing these exercises while you are stuck in traffic can turn a frustrating experience into a meditation in motion and help you deal with other drivers' road rage.

• While watching the television news.

• While on hold during a phone call. With more and more people using call-waiting, it seems like a wonderful new opportunity to Kegel.

• Standing in line at the bank, movies, or at the supermarket.

One of the biggest obstacles to Kegeling is simply forgetting to do it. That is why I recommend buying sticky notes in various bright colors, marking several with a large "K," and placing them in various spots where they can serve as reminders.

HOW OFTEN TO KEGEL

Ideally, Kegel exercises should be performed three times a day, but do not assign yourself such an overly ambitious program that you cannot follow it. You could become discouraged and stop Kegeling altogether.

After a month or two of regular practice, you should feel a marked increase in control over your urine stream, which means that your pelvic muscles have gained strength and tone.

HOW TO KEGEL

There are different types of Kegel exercises. For best results, include each type in every session.

Before you start Kegeling, first practice stopping and starting the flow of urine until you become familiar with your PC muscle and gain some control over it. Another way to determine which muscles need to be contracted is to place two fingers inside the vagina and then press those fingers together by squeezing the vaginal walls shut.

- **Pumps.** Squeeze the PC muscle, hold for three seconds, then relax for three seconds. Repeat as many times as you can, working up to thirty 3-second squeezes at a time.
- **Pulses.** Squeeze and relax the PC muscle quickly, in a fluttering motion. Start slowly at first, aiming for regular contractions rather than speed. Over time, you will be able to do this at a faster, even pace.
- **Bear-downs.** This variation also tones your lower abs. It is done by adding a gentle bearing-down motion to your contraction-relaxation pattern, as if you are having a bowel movement. Hold and release for three seconds at a time, working up to thirty sets. Do not be too forceful; the operative word is "gentle."

A SAMPLE KEGELING SESSION

- Exhale as you give a short squeeze. Squeeze the PC muscle and anal sphincter fifteen to twenty times at approximately one squeeze per second. Make sure that your buttock muscles are not contracting too. It is important to isolate and work only the PC muscle and anal sphincter. Gradually build up to two sets of seventy-five 1-second squeezes per day.
- Squeeze the PC muscle and anal sphincter for a count of three. Relax for three counts. Work up to contracting for ten seconds, and relaxing for ten seconds. Start with two sets of twenty 3-second squeezes each and build up to seventy-five 10-second squeezes.

When you become practiced and toned, add very gentle bear-downs. After releasing the contraction, push down and out gently with your PC muscle and anal sphincter, as if you were having a bowel movement. Start with two sets of twenty bear-downs, and build up to seventy-five bear-downs.

You can work up to 300 Kegel repetitions a day, combining short and long squeezes and bear-downs.

Healthy Stretches

A pliant spine and flexible muscles are the key to eternal youth and health. A flexible lower spine is particularly essential because it helps you enjoy the level of pelvic mobility that maintains optimum circulation. If your spine and pelvis are rigid and tight, energy and blood flow are impeded, and the result is poor hormone balance, gynecological weakness, and conditions such as fibroids.

Many of us suffer from muscular rigidity because we carry around the burden and stress of our problems and worries in our bodies. We have all seen people who walk around slumped over, as if they are bearing the weight of the world on their shoulders and backs. That is how they often feel. Stretching helps release chronically tight musculature so that your energy circulates and flows freely in and out of the pelvic area and your breathing is freed to energize the entire body. Since the blood carries oxygen and nutrients to cells and also removes wastes and toxins, it is easy to see how chronic body tension can lead to poor circulation, compromised health, and the conditions of congestion, stagnation, and hormonal imbalance that lead to fibroids. Stretching can also help relieve stress and stress-associated health problems. This is one reason why massage and various other types of bodywork are so helpful in restoring health. These techniques help soften the armoring that many of us develop in an attempt to keep our problems locked up inside. It is not too much of a leap to recognize that energy stagnation can also develop in the pelvic area after years, even decades, of tightening that area's muscles in an effort to hold back painful emotions and memories. Imagine a pool of stagnant water. No water flows in or out, so stagnation results. It is the same with pelvic congestion. The only way to relieve energy stagnation is to restore balanced energy flow. In fact, fibroids are viewed by traditional Eastern medicine as the end result of stagnated energy. In the absence of free flow, energy solidifies and eventually forms the masses we call fibroids.

DANCING AND HEALTH

The link between dancing and health may not be obvious, but, alone or with a partner, dancing freely—moving wherever the music and your spirit take you—is a tremendously liberating and stress-releasing experience. Put your favorite music on the stereo and let loose. You will probably laugh, maybe even feel a bit embarrassed at first. Do not let that stop you. Dance every day to free your energy and recharge your soul. Belly or Middle Eastern dancing, all styles of African dancing, some forms of East Indian dancing, reggae dancing from Jamaica, and soca and calypso dancing from Trinidad and Tobago are particularly beneficial because they help make your torso more mobile. All these dance styles help soften the muscular armor that causes pelvic energy to stagnate.

Take dance classes. Or buy a videotape and dance along. Or go to an African, Middle Eastern, Indian, or Caribbean dance club. You are not just having fun! You are learning to "wind your waistline," as Caribbean people call it. That is, you are recovering your torso's natural flexibility along with your health, and you are dissolving many years' worth of stagnated, solidified chi.

BASIC BODY STRETCH

One of life's greatest pleasures is a good, long stretch. You can actually feel your body release tension. You automatically inhale and exhale more deeply, oxygenate your blood more thoroughly, and get rid of toxins. A limber and flexible body is a healthy, fit body, and no workout is complete without stretching every part to keep muscles from shortening and becoming stiff.

If you add a long, loud sigh to your exhalations, you will discover that the benefits are even greater. Your body grows even more relaxed, your capacity to stretch increases, and your mind calms.

- Lie on your back, arms comfortably extended over your head and a little out to the sides, legs extended and relaxed slightly to each side.
- Push your heels forward, at the same time pressing your lower spine against the floor.
- Press and release your spine a few times to limber it up.

Now that your lower spine has enjoyed a little stretch, press it against the floor again, at the same time stretching your arms away from your head and your legs away from your hips, extending your heels. Be sure to keep all four limbs on the floor. Inhale as you stretch, and feel your muscles grow more flexible with each exhalation.

SITTING FORWARD STRETCH

Another stretch to increase your spine's flexibility.

- Sit comfortably on the floor, legs extended straight in front of you, a little less than hip-width apart.
- Support your weight with hands placed on either side of your hips in order to lift your buttocks off the floor. Make sure that you are seated forward on your hips and that your spine is straight.
- Stretching from the hip joints rather than your back, lean forward, keeping the back straight. At the same time, extend your heels forward to maximize the stretch. Think of bringing the lower abdomen closer to the thighs.

Do not worry about how far you bend. Hold at the point of your farthest stretch and take ten slow, deep breaths. You should feel the back of the calves and hamstrings give way a little more.

YOGA

Traditional Eastern healers and philosophers understood the profound connection between physical exercise and optimal health of body, mind, and spirit for many centuries before Westerners began to catch on. The practice of yoga from India and virtually all the Taoist exercises from ancient China were designed specifically to help their practitioners enjoy youthful energy, passion, and health throughout their lives. I committed myself to a life with yoga after being inspired by a seventy-six year-old yoga instructor named Jack England. Jack began doing yoga after he suffered a severe back injury at the age of fifty. He now teaches yoga every day to groups of much younger people who hang on every word he delivers as he stretches and twists his body into unimaginable poses. Here is one of Jack's favorite nuggets of wisdom: "You don't get old and then stiff, you get stiff and *then* you are old." If you start stretching and practicing yoga now, you will restore your body to the level of flexibility and health you enjoyed when you were a child.

"Yoga," which means the union of body and mind through breath, developed in India three to five thousand years ago. Many of the newer holistic western exercise and bodywork systems described later in this chapter draw from the bottomless well of yogic body-mind philosophy.

HATHA YOGA

Hatha yoga, the form of yoga with which Westerners are most familiar, focuses on energizing and toning the body, and making it flexible. It consists of physical postures and breathing exercises that enhance general health. The benefits to gynecological health are especially powerful. Establishing a regular daily or weekly yoga practice is one of the most effective ways you can secure your health and help your hormone system normalize.

The main differences between yoga and Western exercise are: yoga emphasizes inner, along with outer, health, and there is no element of competition. The breath is used to promote well-being and self-awareness and to facilitate holding various postures. Unlike Western exercises, which can exhaust you, yoga never drains your energy. After performing yoga exercises, you feel more vital and balanced. Yoga also improves endurance and flexibility and gives you stronger, more flexible spine and joints. As the body becomes more flexible, so do the mind and spirit. This is why regular yoga practice calms the mind and spirit. When you give in to the pose, you are focused in the present moment, which is the objective of any meditation practice. Remember the hit comedy movie *City Slickers*? When Billy Crystal's character asks Jack Palance's mysterious cowboy to tell him the secret of life, Palance raises a single finger and smiles. Crystal's character spends the rest of the movie trying to figure out what Palance means. He never realizes that the single finger means that we should do only one thing at a time. In other words, do not eat while driving, read while walking, and so on. A regular yoga practice helps train your focus on one thing at a time, which helps you conduct your life at a calmer, more focused and meditative state.

Although yoga teachers recommend practicing yoga for at least one hour, several times a week, a little yoga goes a long way. You can practice the following simple yoga postures (also called "asanas") almost anywhere, and in a very brief period of time.

If possible, yoga should be practiced in loose clothing and at least two hours after a meal. Remember: Yoga is not a competitive sport but a wonderful gift to yourself. Do the postures at your own pace, never forcing your body into any position it is not ready to assume. I recommend taking yoga classes so you can be monitored and corrected, but these easy, simple postures can be done on your own.

BASIC EASTERN BREATH

Most of us Westerners are shallow breathers who use only one-seventh to one-third of our lung capacity, robbing ourselves not only of oxygen but also of the life-force energy we need for good health and healing. The "basic breath" is common to all Eastern disciplines. Virtually all eastern disciplines begin with the breath because it carries into and out of the body the life-force energy, or "chi," that animates us and connects us to the greater whole. This is important to those of us who do not breathe deeply enough to energize ourselves fully and ensure sufficient circulation in the pelvic organs and glands. This deep belly breath also pushes down your diaphragm (the muscular separation between the lungs and the abdominal cavity), giving a "massage" to the organs in the abdominal cavity. When we fill the pelvic girdle with fresh oxygen, we bring energy, warmth, and life to the uterus, ovaries, and other pelvic organs and glands.

If you can control your breath, you control your energy, which means that you will enjoy limitless benefits. As you breathe during this exercise, visualize your pelvis as a balloon that inflates with air on inhalation and deflates on exhalation. This deep breathing pattern will wake up, energize, and strengthen all your pelvic organs and glands.

For most Eastern breathing exercises, breathe in and out through the nostrils only, unless otherwise instructed.

- Lie on your back with knees bent, feet about shoulder-width apart and planted on the floor. Make sure the small of the back is relaxed against the floor. You may want to place a rolled-up towel or pillow under your knees to help the abdomen and back relax completely.
- Place the right hand gently on your lower abdomen and the left on your chest. Inhale, slowly, evenly, and deeply, so that the right hand rises. The left hand should stay still. As you exhale, the right hand should lower.

- Close your eyes to help you tune in to your breath and become aware of how energy is filling and energizing your body. See the breath entering the space containing the pelvic organs. Know that it is bringing healing, radiant light in and taking toxins and wastes out.

- Take several long, slow, deep breaths, trying to expand your abdomen a little more with each inhalation. Never force or hold your breath.

- Now imagine that each inhalation is filling your entire torso. The top is your neck and the bottom is the perineum (the area between the anus and urethra—the opening of the urinary tract). The sides include the circumference of the rib cage, the stomach, and back.

- Inhale, first filling the bottom, then the top, and finally the entire circumference. Feel your rib cage expand as you inhale. Feel your genital area fill with energy and a deliciously alive sensation. Allow the space between the shoulder blades to relax open.

- As you continue taking long inhalations and exhalations, allow your breath to travel into your legs and arms, filling your limbs with vital energy, all the way down to the tips of the fingers and toes.

This breath may feel awkward at first, but after you have practiced it regularly for a while, it will become easy, familiar, and automatic.

Great times to practice are in the morning before you get out of bed and start your day, and at night, before you drop off to sleep. The Basic Eastern Breath is a wonderful way to shed tension at the end of the day. It also eases insomnia.

Once you are comfortable with this breathing exercise while lying down, practice it in a sitting position, always making sure that the abdomen is moving out with each inhalation and in with each exhalation, and that the chest stays still. You can use the basic breath any time you find yourself stuck in traffic, on line, or in a boring or stressful situation.

Experiment with this breath. First breathe in the typically shallow fashion, raising your shoulders as you take in short, shallow inhalations. Sense how tense and irritable you become. Next, perform the deep belly breathing of the Basic Eastern Breath. Notice how much calmer and more relaxed you feel. Now you have a quick, easy tool to help you cope with daily stress. Any time you notice yourself tensing up, simply take several deep, long belly breaths. You will be amazed how much easier it becomes to cope with life's challenges.

This is also the basic breathing pattern you will use in every yoga asana, as well as in the Taoist exercises that follow.

Alternate Nostril Breathing

This breathing exercise calms, purifies, and energizes, and puts you in touch with the life-force energy flowing through your body. You deliberately slow and balance the breath in order to relieve stress on the heart and central nervous system and steady the metabolism. As you know, relieving stress and steadying your metabolism help bring your hormones into balance.

Find a quiet place to be alone, such as your office or a bathroom. Sit with your back straight so that your lungs will have maximum room to expand. This is also a great exercise for morning or night, and it is an especially effective way to mark the transition between work and home, so you feel more relaxed and enjoy a good night's sleep.

- Exhale completely, contracting and drawing in the abdominal muscles to force air steadily from your lungs.
- Close the right nostril with the right thumb, then slowly inhale through the left nostril. Do not overinflate your lungs.
- When the lungs are filled to comfortable capacity, also close the left nostril, using the fourth (ring) finger and your

pinky finger. Fold the index and middle fingers into the palm to keep them out of the way.

• When you have filled your lungs and closed off both nostrils, hold the breath inside the lungs for as long as it is comfortable.

When you first start to practice this breath, the period of retention will not be long, but it will increase as you proceed.

• As soon as you feel any discomfort, open the right nostril, and—keeping the left nostril closed with the ring and pinky fingers—slowly exhale through the right nostril.

• Inhale through the left nostril and repeat the above steps.

The three phases—exhalation→inhalation-block→switch—constitute a round (which always begins and ends on an exhalation). A round is one complete cycle.

If you are a first-timer, try six to ten rounds for three to five minutes. Make sure the breath flows silently, a sign that it is not being forced. After a few rounds, exhale and inhale to the count of four. As you gain control, make your exhalations twice as long as your inhalations, and gradually increase the total number of rounds to twenty or more.

If you have time, practice this exercise several times a day. Otherwise, once a day, or whenever you feel stressed, is fine.

HATHA YOGA POSTURES (ASANAS)

Even if you have only a few free moments, just one or two yoga postures will lift your spirits and energy instantly. Focus on your inner body as you do these postures by continuously performing the Basic Eastern Breath.

Relaxation Pose

Lie on your back on the floor, your feet about two feet apart, arms extended slightly away from your sides. If you feel any discomfort in your lower back, bend the knees and bring them together. Or roll up a pillow and place it under your knees so your lower back relaxes into the floor and your abdomen softens.

- Close your eyes and begin the Basic Eastern Breath. Turn your attention to the breath and follow its rhythms. Do not try to change anything; simply observe it. Is it slowing down? Is it becoming more shallow? Are the exhalations longer than the inhalations?
- If you drop off to sleep for a while, that's okay. You can even practice this exercise in bed at night to carry you off to dreamland.

Whether you fall asleep or not, you will come out of this pose feeling refreshed and energized. For those of you who find a daytime nap disorienting, the relaxation pose is a great substitute, especially when you have little time. I have found that five to fifteen minutes of this pose combined with the Basic Eastern Breath is extremely refreshing and energizing. When I was still delivering babies and missing several nights' sleep each week, I used this meditative belly breathing to get me through many days at the office.

The Mountain Pose

This basic posture tones and energizes the entire body. It also helps you feel grounded so you have a stronger sense of being "rooted." This gives you a more powerful, positive sense of self that better equips you to take charge of your health and healing.

- Stand with bare feet (if possible) shoulder-width apart. Focus your awareness on the sensation of being planted on the floor.
- Lift and spread your toes, then try to bring them back to the floor one at a time, starting with the small toe and progressing to the big toe. This will give you a wider foundation.

• Starting with your ankles and focusing on your spine, lengthen your body from the feet up, all the while maintaining that strong connection to the floor through your feet. Reach up from your ankles to your knees, then from knees to hip sockets, from hips to waist, waist to shoulders. Drop your shoulders as you lengthen your neck, tilt your chin slightly in, and stretch the top of your head toward the ceiling.

• Relax your shoulders, letting them "melt" downward, away from your ears. Allow your arms to hang loosely, fingers relaxed and soft. Like a mountain, you are rooted in the earth and reaching for the sky.

Standing Forward Bend

This posture helps shed stiffness, rigidity, and tension by gently stretching the entire back of the body, thus increasing your energy level, dissolving energy blockages, and increasing energy flow. Assume the Mountain Pose stance.

• Bend your elbows and place your hands on the front crease between your thighs and hips.

• Bending slowly and steadily from the hip sockets while keeping a straight back, lower your torso. At the same time, slide your hands down the fronts of your legs. Bend as far forward as you can while maintaining a straight back.

• Hold the posture and keep performing the Basic Eastern Breath.

• Now, allow your back to relax loosely and let your head and neck dangle freely. Make sure that your neck, shoulders, and arms are relaxed.

• Hold the pose, remembering to breathe, as long as you are comfortable.

• When you are ready, come out of the pose by bringing your torso back up slowly, back rounded, hands on your hip sockets, until you are back in the Mountain Pose.

Seated Forward Bend

This is an alternative posture you can do at your desk in your office or from any other seat. Because your head goes below your heart, it receives an increased blood supply that energizes you mentally and physically.

- Sit in a chair about halfway forward on the seat, feet on the floor, knees about shoulder-width apart.
- Inhale, then exhale as you allow your torso to drop forward slowly between your knees and place both hands—one at a time—on the floor between your feet.
- Hang forward, neck and shoulders relaxed and completely free of support.
- Use the Basic Eastern Breath to inhale life-force energy into any area of your body that feels tight or stagnated. As you exhale, see stress leaving your body. Stay in the posture as long as you are comfortable.
- Come up slowly, bracing one hand against a thigh for support. Sit for a moment or two with your eyes closed, doing the Basic Eastern Breath and moving your awareness through your body to sense which parts have relaxed and which parts are still tense. Breathe into those tense areas, then let the tension go on your exhalations.

Shoulder and Neck Yoga Stretches

These stress-releasing stretches can be done anywhere—sitting or standing—and they are a wonderful way either to end the day or prepare for your healing meditation and visualization sessions. Remember not to slump. Keep your spine long, as you straighten and lengthen from its base.

- Lift your shoulders and roll them in 360-degree circles, to the front, up toward your ears, then back and down. Keep breathing, sending each inhalation into a different tense spot and feeling it let go as you exhale.

- Repeat the circle several times, then do several rolls in the opposite direction.
- Keep doing this until your shoulders feel soft and relaxed.
- Now, stretch your neck by slowly dropping your chin toward your chest. Let your head hang free, as you breathe tension out of the tight spots.
- Slowly bring your head back to center, then drop it gradually to the right side, so that your right ear is leaning over your right shoulder. Keep breathing as each exhalation gently increases the stretch. Repeat on the opposite side. Never let your head drop straight back; this can damage your cervical spine.

The Butterfly

The yoga poses that I just described stretch, relax, and energize your inner and outer body. The Butterfly has an even more direct benefit on gynecological health because it opens and softens the hip joints and stretches and tones the inner thighs. This pose also increases circulation in the pelvic area and helps relieve painful cramping associated with fibroids and other hormone imbalance–related conditions.

- Sit on the floor and bend your knees. Bring the soles of your feet together, allowing your knees to drop open gently to either side of the body.
- Take hold of your feet, and draw them as close to you as possible, keeping your spine tall and shoulders relaxed.
- Hold this pose and practice the Basic Eastern Breath, visualizing energy going to your inner thighs, pelvic joints, and pelvic organs. Allow the stretch to gently increase with each long, even exhalation. If you feel any discomfort, sigh as you exhale to help release it.
- Hold this pose as long as possible, filling your pelvic area with purifying air and energy and exhaling your inner thighs and hip joints further into the stretch.

TANTRIC YOGA PELVIS SWINGS

Many Western bodywork therapies that aim to free energy flow blocked by chronically contracted torso muscles were inspired by the following exercise.

Variation One: On All Fours ("Cat–Cow")

• Place your knees and palms on the floor, fingers facing forward and spread apart, thighs and arms at right angles to the floor. Your neck should extend straight from your spine, neither tipping upward nor hanging downward.

• As you inhale deeply and slowly into your belly, tip your head and buttocks up, arching your back. Your belly should expand as it fills with air, and your pelvic girdle relaxes and opens.

• Exhale slowly, at the same time tightening your buttocks and tipping your pelvis forward and under. Your back should round. Feel your pelvis muscles contract and tighten.

• Repeat this action: rhythmically inhaling, arching your back and opening your pelvis; then exhaling as you round your back while tightening your pelvis and buttocks muscles.

Variation Two: Standing

• Stand with legs about hip-width apart. Feel your feet planted on the floor, body weight evenly distributed between the heels and balls of your feet.

• Lift your toes, spread them apart, then let them float down to the floor. Feel how the bottoms of your feet, including the toes, support your weight.

• Let your knees be loose and slightly flexed. Rock slightly back and forth between the balls of your feet and the heels. Settle into a strong, grounded stance.

• As you inhale air into your belly, let your pelvis swing easily backward from the "hinge" of the hips. Do not move your waist or legs, just the pelvis.

- As you exhale, tighten your abs to expel the air slowly and steadily. At the same time, contract the buttocks and push the pelvis into a forward tilt.
- Use your arms to help you. Allow them to dangle loosely at your sides, swinging backward with the pelvis as you inhale, then swinging forward with the pelvis as you exhale.
- If you feel tight and "locked"—that is, if your pelvis is unable to make these movements easily—keep practicing. Observe your movements and correct them in front of a mirror. Do this exercise regularly and you are sure to loosen up.

Practice this exercise every day for five to ten minutes.

- When you are able to synchronize your breathing with the pelvic rocking and arm swings, bring in your PC muscle. As you inhale, allow your genitals to "open" and fully relax, imagining that they are filling with life-giving energy. As you exhale, contract or "lock" the PC muscle and anus as you would for a Kegel contraction, to prevent the energy you have gathered from leaking out.

Tao Exercises

Until quite recently, many Taoist exercises and techniques were practiced only by Chinese holy men and nobility and were kept secret from the rest of the world. Although Taoist exercises have not achieved the popularity of yoga here in the West, they share many features.

Both yoga and the Tao are about the art of self-healing through cultivating and controlling life-force energy. Some Taoist practices are even more effective at gathering and increasing life-force energy in the pelvic area. Special Taoist postures give the dedicated practitioner an astounding degree of control over her body, especially the ability to build and transform energy into a healing force.

Taoists cultivate pelvic energy for greater health and spiritual awareness because all the body's energy currents (also known as acupuncture meridians) pass through the pelvis. If the pelvic area is blocked, you lose valuable life-energy, and all your organs and glands—even your brain—suffer. Most of us experience an abundance of life-force energy only in our youth. We do not know how to preserve and channel this energy, let alone how to restore and multiply it.

The SAD program, alcohol, drugs, smoking, and other abuses that offer only fleeting satisfaction gradually wear us out. By middle or old age, the pelvic and rectal muscles have weakened, sagged, and loosened, allowing vital energy to drain out of the body, and making the person more prone to disease and dysfunction, including the development of fibroid tumors.

Increasingly, though, many relatively young people are suffering from loss of vital life-force energy. Taoist exercises are among the best remedies for the all-too-common modern-day symptoms of chronic fatigue, lack of sexual desire, impotence, infertility, lower abdominal inflammatory conditions, PMS, menstrual disorders, fibroids, and other debilitating conditions, even for depression and other negative emotional states.

Taoist exercises strengthen and revitalize the pelvic organs and hormone glands by literally increasing and concentrating energy in that area. Exercises are designed to build up energy, then literally pump that energy from the ovaries to the uterus and vagina, across the perineum, and up the spine. As life-force energy travels, it heals the nerves—all the way up to the brain. After it circulates through the brain, it is directed down the front of the body—healing other organs and glands in its path. Finally, it settles in the navel area, where it is stored. This circle of energy is accomplished through a combination of breath control, visualization, and flexing of the perineal muscles, which include the PC muscle, the vaginal walls, and the anal spincter—exactly the way you contract your PC muscle when Kegeling.

Unless otherwise instructed, use the Basic Eastern Breath while performing all Taoist exercises.

FIRE BELLY

This exercise helps stoke the "fire," or energy, contained in the area from about one inch above the pubic bone to about an inch and a half below the navel—the power center for all our body functions and activities. Practice this breath regularly and you will have much more energy and strength. You will also help normalize your hormone levels. This exercise is best performed nude or wearing loose natural-fiber clothing.

- Stand, feet apart and knees slightly flexed, or sit on the edge of a chair, back straight, feet on the floor.
- Rub the palms of your hands together briskly, until they are hot.
- Make gentle circular motions on your lower abdomen with your left hand, covering the area from just below the navel to just above the pubic bone. Do this clockwise several times.
- Rub your palms together to heat them up again.
- Use your right hand to massage the same area several times, this time in a counterclockwise motion.

Make as many circles as you wish, making sure to rub an equal number of times in each direction.

THE KIDNEY STIMULATOR

The Kidney Stimulator strengthens the kidneys, adrenals, and the rest of the glandular system, increasing hormone production and balance and improving general strength and energy. It even helps relieve lower back pain, cures infertility, and keeps skin smooth and beautiful.

- Sit or lie down comfortably. Rub the palms together briskly until they are very warm.
- Place your palms on the small of your back as you tilt your

upper body slightly forward. Feel and visualize the energy flowing from your hands into your kidneys and adrenals.

- Massage the small of your back by rubbing up and down and then rubbing in a circular motion.
- Now, make a loose fist and softly pummel the small of your back for a few seconds.
- Repeat the rubbing and pummeling three times.

THE DEER

This basic but powerfully effective Taoist exercise increases and balances hormone gland secretions and boosts energy levels. When your hormone glands function at optimum levels, you feel fully energized, toned, and rejuvenated and your body can create its own healing miracles. The Deer is also based on the principle that the foundation of lifelong good health and vitality is having strong, toned vaginal and anal muscles. When these muscles are strong, they benefit the uterus and ovaries and help prevent many common gynecological maladies, including fibroid conditions. The Deer also helps prevent and cure hemorrhoids and relieves the symptoms of menopause.

Practice the Deer after bathing and in the nude.

- Sit on the floor, a couch, or bed, and draw the heel of one foot up against your groin so that it presses against the opening of your vagina and clitoris. If your heel will not reach, place a hard round object, such as child's ball, against the area, until you feel a gentle, pleasurably stimulating pressure.
- Rub your palms together briskly to build up heat, then cover your breasts with your hands and feel the heat penetrate every cell.
- Now, rub your breasts gently but firmly in outward, circular motions. Move the right hand in a clockwise direction, the left in a counterclockwise direction. Taoists recommend doing this for a minimum of 36 circles and a maximum of 306 circles,

but you can circle as many times as you wish. Just be sure to circle in each direction an equal number of times. This outward massage clears congestion, preventing and even curing lumps and cysts.

• Rub your hands together briskly again. Reverse directions, rubbing your breasts in an inward, circular motion to stimulate them (right hand, counterclockwise; left hand, clockwise). This direction increases their size and firmness.

• Now, tighten your anal and vaginal muscles as if you were doing a Kegel contraction, and hold it as long as comfortable. Relax, then repeat.

After weeks of regular practice, you should be able to hold the contraction for a longer period. When you gain more control, you will be able do the Kegel contractions, or energy locks, at the same time you are rubbing your breasts.

When you become completely comfortable with the Deer, you can go on to moving the energy you have gathered in a circle through your entire body with the following exercise.

ENERGY CIRCLE
• Practice the Deer to build up energy.
• Inhale and feel the energy gather.
• Exhale and feel the energy move down from your uterus and ovaries to your vagina. Use as many inhalations and exhalations as you need to feel the energy move.
• Now as you inhale, arch your lower back and move your buttocks back in a pelvic tilting movement.
• Exhale and allow your back and hips to return to resting position. This creates a pumping action that moves the energy. Feel the energy move across the perineum each time you pump. Again, use as many breaths as you need to move the energy.
• Inhale as you tilt your hips, then exhale and relax back to a resting position to pump the energy to the base of your spine.

- Keep pumping the energy with pelvic tilts and your breathing, moving it in stages up your spine to your brain.
- See the energy circle through your brain. Now, allow it to move with each exhalation—down your forehead, nose, mouth, throat, and then down the front of your body, healing and revitalizing every organ and gland in its path.

This exercise may seem difficult, but all you need is practice and patience. Even if you cannot move the energy at first, and, then, only in a limited way, you will still reap this exercise's many wonderful health benefits.

Acupressure

Both acupuncture and acupressure are based on a detailed energy map of the human body that locates the precise channels (known as meridians) through which life-force energy travels in order to bring energy through to each body part. All diseases, weakness, and dysfunctions—including those that create fibroid conditions—are thought to be caused by blockages of life-force energy that cause either energy stagnation or energy deficiency in various organ and gland systems.

Acupressure, which is called "shiatsu" by the Japanese, consists of finger pressure applied to specific points along those meridians in order to unblock life-force energy. The result is stimulated circulation, relief from pain, and revitalization of your entire being. Since all traditional eastern healing systems view the body as an integrated whole, virtually any blockage in the body will have an adverse effect on gynecological health and hormone balance.

It may be more pleasurable to have someone work on you, but you can also do it yourself anytime, at your convenience, and you do not have to pay a single cent.

HOW TO APPLY SELF-ACUPRESSURE

Always use firm pressure to stimulate the body's natural curative abilities. It will hurt a bit—especially if a particular point really needs treatment. But this slight pain should feel "sweet," as it also brings energy flow and release.

Use your thumb, finger, palm, the side of a hand, or your knuckles to apply the pressure. Some professional acupressure practitioners even use their feet and elbows.

Use prolonged, steady pressure; three minutes per point is ideal.

POINTS FOR GYNECOLOGICAL VITALITY

• Sea of Vitality

Location: Altogether, this treatment includes four points located on the lower back, two and four finger-widths away from the spine on either side, at waist level.

Benefits: Relieves lower backaches, fatigue, reproductive and gynecological problems.

• Bubbling Springs

Location: One point on each foot, in the center of the sole of the foot, at the base of the ball of the foot, between the two pads.

Benefits: Relieves PMS and menopausal symptoms.

• Bigger Stream

Location: One point on each foot, midway between the inside anklebone and the Achilles tendon, on the back of the ankle.

Benefits: Relieves menstrual irregularity and fatigue.

Caution: Do not use this point after the third month of pregnancy.

• Three Mile Point

Location: Four finger-widths below each kneecap, one finger-width on the outside of each shinbone. If you are on the correct spot, a muscle should flex under your finger, as you move your foot up and down.

Benefits: Strengthens entire body, especially the muscles, and boosts the entire gynecological system.

Again, the key to establishing a regular, health-enhancing exercise program is to take a gradual approach. Do not assign yourself such an overly ambitious exercise schedule that it becomes a struggle you may give up. These exercises should become a pleasurable experience that you want to practice regularly. The way to success with exercise, as with so many other activities, is through consistent practice.

8

The Threat of Environmental Toxins—Xenobiotics

Not war, but a plethora of man-made things is threatening to strangle us, suffocate us, bury us, in the debris and by-products of our technically inventive age.

—RACHEL CARSON, *Silent Spring*

In Chapter 2 you learned about xenoestrogens, the chemicals in pesticides, insecticides, and other substances that are part and parcel of our modern times. Xenoestrogens are in our food, water, plastics, cleaning substances, and just about everything else. For some, these chemicals represent the fruits of cutting-edge science, but from a holistic health point of view, they are our worst nightmare. When it comes to animal and human reproductive health, xenoestrogens are a full-fledged disaster.

These chemicals act as "false" estrogens in the body, replacing healthy, natural estrogens on hormone receptor sites and disrupting the entire hormonal chain of command. The damage includes a variety of menstrual dysfunctions, PMS, fibroids, and worse. Let us take a closer look at these toxins and other common, everyday poisons in order to understand more fully how they affect our health and the development of fibroids.

The Toxic Threat

In the fifties, Rachel Carson's groundbreaking *Silent Spring* sounded an alarm. Hers was the first book to tackle the controversial subject of environmental poisons. It detailed the destructive impact on our environment of a growing and widespread use of pesticides and insecticides. She reported on the thinning and breaking apart of birds' eggshells, reduced fertility, and other worrisome alterations in wild animal life. She warned that fish and other forms of life in our lakes and streams were dying for no discernible reason. These were the warning signs, she wrote, of imminent and dire consequences to human health and to the earth itself. The cause, she stated, was the unbridled use of xenoestrogens, hormone-disrupting chemical agents. Carson stressed the fact that the only solution was to limit the use of these toxins.

Unfortunately, few people heeded Carson's alarm, and her warnings remain as urgent today as they were half a century ago. Vested-interest groups such as industrial farming corporations, international chemical companies, and other agencies continue to lobby strenuously for the continued use of toxic chemicals. We know more today than ever before about the link between reproductive dysfunction and environmental poisons, yet pesticides, insecticides, and other harmful chemicals are still ubiquitous. These toxins and their profoundly adverse effects on human health are still hotly debated, with threatened industries sparing no expense to counter the claims made by scientists and other advocates for the environment and our health.

✦ Joan's Story

Joan, a thirty-five-year-old journalist, suffered from subserous and intramural fibroids. Besides abnormally heavy periods, a profound sense of fatigue was robbing Joan of any enjoyment in life. Even worse, her symptoms had worsened dramatically in the few weeks before she consulted me, threatening to jeopardize her livelihood. She simply lacked the energy to chase down a news story at any time of day or night.

Joan was quite sophisticated about holistic medicine and had tried treating herself with herbs and supplements. Yet, no matter how many vitamins, minerals, and other supplements she swallowed, it was still a struggle for her to get out of bed.

My preliminary workup revealed nothing wrong, so I decided to do a hair analysis. This test analyzes a sample of hair taken from close to the scalp for excessive or deficient levels of various minerals. The test results provided a possible answer to Joan's problems: high levels of toxic mercury (Hg) in her body. I placed Joan on a program to remove the mercury from her system. After a month or so, Joan had recovered enough energy to follow a more comprehensive fibroid-healing program. Another few months passed, and Joan felt almost fully recovered and able to engage completely in her life and work.

Most people who are affected by modern-day toxins do not even realize that this is why they are struggling through their days, always feeling tired and sick. Nor does anyone know for certain the full extent of the damage caused by chemical sensitivities. We know that among the most dangerous culprits are pesticides and insecticides (including the most infamous insecticide of them all, dichlorodiphenyltrichloroethane, better known as DDT), petrochemicals, polychlorinated biphenyls (PCBs), and chlorinated hydrocarbons.

Less Obvious, but Just as Toxic

Other toxins are less obvious villains. Evidence suggests that the fluoride in drinking water; the chlorine in swimming pools, public water supplies, and household cleansers; and the bromides used in many baked goods in the form of baking powder are disrupting thyroid gland function by interfering with how the body uses iodine.

Fluoride, chlorine, iodine, and bromine form the halogen family of elements, and each member of that family can substitute for the other in your body. Yet your body cannot make use of any type of halogen except for iodine. If fluoride, bromides, or chlorine beat the iodine to your body's iodine receptor sites, not enough iodine will get into your body tissues to ensure a smooth-functioning thyroid gland. You have learned about the intricate hormonal web that ties the menstrual cycle to virtually every other body function. The endocrine system "speaks" to the nervous system, the immune system, the gastrointestinal system, and the rest of the body, and then they all engage in dialogue in this complex web of interaction. The downside of all the interrelatedness is that any problem in one part will inevitably lead to problems somewhere else. Disruption in thyroid gland function can cause problems with your reproductive system through this hormonal web.

THE SAD TOXIC THREAT

You know that the foods included in the Standard American Diet (SAD) are not good for you, in part because of their poor nutritional content. For example, your diet must include enough foods rich in vitamin B_6, because that vitamin is essential for the liver, so it can metabolize and clear excess hormones. Recent studies show that vitamin B_6 is also important for the effective attachment of estrogens to the appropriate receptor site. If your diet is deficient in B_6 you can develop the estrogen-dominant state that leads to fibroids and other hormone-dependent conditions.

But the SAD program poses even more dangers than nutritional deficiencies, including one related to vitamin B_6. The SAD diet may be empty of nutrition, but it is full of a group of chemicals called hydrazines that are used in food colorings (tartrazine), herbicides, and other common food stuffs. Hydrazines actually "look like" vitamin B_6 to the body, so this group of chemicals is accepted by the body as B_6. Unfortunately, hydrazines and other vitamin lookalikes do not function in the body as the real nutrients do. Hydrazines actually block the beneficial and necessary B_6 effect that is essential to maintain hormone balance. Many experts also believe that hydrazine consumption may be responsible, at least in part, for the current epidemic in such otherwise inexplicable conditions as carpal tunnel syndrome, attention deficit disorder, and kidney stones, as well as hormone-dependent conditions such as PMS and fibroid tumors.

THE HEAVY METAL TOXIC THREAT

Toxicity from heavy metals is another problem currently afflicting countless people with a weird array of symptoms that include fatigue, muscle aches and pains, mood swings, depression, and hormone-dependent conditions. Aluminum is a heavy metal found everywhere in our environment—in antiperspirants, antacids, and many foods, such as commercially prepared cheese. Although authorities assure us that the body does not absorb aluminum through the skin, recent studies suggest the opposite. Aluminum *is* absorbed through the skin, then makes its way to the bones and brain, where it increases the risk for both osteoporosis and Alzheimer's disease.

In one study, patients who were scheduled to have operations on their bones or brains were separated into two groups. One group used an antiperspirant containing aluminum and the other group did not. When the surgeries were performed, the group that used the products containing aluminum showed increases of the metal in both brain and bone. We do not yet understand the full implications of this finding, but with the increases in Alzheimer's disease and osteoporosis, it seems prudent to avoid exposure to aluminum as much as possible.

Just leaving tomato sauce in the tin can after you have opened it will cause an appreciable amount of the tin to leach into the sauce. The tomato sauce's acidity acts in partnership with exposure to the air to actually dissolve the tin. Using aluminum foil to cover any acidic food creates a similar risk, because that acid causes the foil to erode so aluminum is absorbed into the food. Have you ever wrapped a slice of pizza in aluminum foil, put it into the refrigerator, then taken it out the next day and found holes in the aluminum foil? Where do you suppose the missing aluminum has gone? You now have a slice with cheese *and aluminum*. Another precaution against aluminum toxicity is to avoid cooking with aluminum pots and pans. Many experts believe that the heating process allows the aluminum to leach into your food.

Other common substances we encounter every day that have been proven harmful to gynecological health include lead, cadmium, and mercury. One of the most common ways in which people become contaminated with mercury is by eating freshwater fish. This is why holistic health experts advocate eating only deep-sea cold-water fish. If you eat from lower on the food chain, you also avoid fish higher on the sea life food chain that have more elevated amounts of mercury and other toxins. Another major source of mercury toxicity is dental amalgams. If mercury toxicity seems to be your problem, ask your dentist to avoid mercury fillings and use some of the newer, less toxic substances.

SICK BUILDING SYNDROME

Yet another big part of this toxic picture are the chemical building products used to construct the modern buildings that also lack windows that open to let in fresh air. They have caused a widespread malady called "sick building syndrome." All these products outgas chemicals that enter our bodies through our lungs, nose, mouth, and skin. Once they are inside us, they exert many negative and horrific effects.

Toxins and Hormones

The pollutants we have discussed and many others are all xenoestrogenic. In fact, they bind even more strongly to your estrogen receptor sites than do natural hormones. They also last longer in your body, where they exert strong and inappropriate effects for a long period, giving them plenty of time to wreak havoc on your gynecological and overall health. Your body attempts to rid itself of these toxins, but the detoxification system can make the situation even more dire by creating stronger and more detrimental metabolites of these compounds that the body is not used to handling and eliminating.

Research confirms that the toxic threat is linked to the widespread increase in such hormone-dependent problems as fibrocystic breast conditions, PMS, ovarian and uterine cancers, polycystic ovarian disease, fertility problems, endometriosis, cervical dysplasia, autoimmune diseases like systemic lupus erythematosus, and, of course, fibroid tumors.

Females are not the only gender affected. Remember those Everglades alligators with abnormally tiny penises? Well, human males are also being affected. No one has reported a widespread reduction in penis size, but one has to wonder about the current glut of ads for penis enlargement surgery and the growing concern over impotence. (Just check the sales figures on Viagra.) We do know for certain that sperm counts are steadily lowering. I told you in Chapter 2 that during my gynecology residency in the seventies, the lower limit for normal sperm count was in the vicinity of 60 million per milliliter. Today, the acceptable lower normal limit is 20 million, only one-third of the previously accepted level! I find it astonishing that instead of launching an urgent quest for the causes of this dramatically lower sperm count, the government of the United States, in all its wisdom, has simply lowered the acceptable "normal" value. Many scientific experts point the finger at environmental toxins. It is clear that these are the prime suspects, at least in large part, for lowered sperm counts. They are also the main culprits behind the increase in such serious male hormone–dependent diseases as prostate and testicular cancer.

TOXIC MEDIA

Some research even suggests that chemical toxins are only one part of a much larger toxic picture. The Niagara of media messages that assaults us on a daily basis is another serious type of pollution. This toxic overstimulation exerts a destructive effect on the brain's limbic system. If you remember, the hormonal chain of command starts with the limbic brain, so anything that adversely effects that essential part of the hormonal web will disturb hormone production and balance and possibly lead to fibroids and other disease conditions. The culprit can be a heavy metal ingested in a meal, a toxic chlorinated hydrocarbon absorbed through our skin from fresh laundry, or a vicious scene on the six o'clock news that scrambles our limbic brain signals. The toxic input we receive from the environment through any of our five senses is passed on, then circulated through our bodies via the interlocking web of the psycho-neuro-endocrine system.

I know the picture that I have painted about the dangers of our modern world looks grim. There is good news, though. You can do much to avoid these dangerous pollutants and cleanse them from your body.

✦ Connie's Story

Connie came to see me after consulting with several gynecologists. Each one had recommended some sort of surgical procedure for her fibroid condition. Connie was not ready for the surgeon's knife, so she was eager and motivated to try out out the less invasive treatments I recommended.

For the previous several months, her periods had been extremely profuse and painful. Connie was used to heavy, crampy menstrual periods, but now they were getting even worse. "I feel fat, like a mess, for two whole weeks before my period," Connie told me. "And whenever my husband and I make love, he can't even touch my breasts without me screaming. They're that tender." Worst of all, Connie's moods were becoming erratic. One moment, she would be on the verge of tears about a minor glitch in her day. The next moment, she would be so overwhelmed with rage that she believed she could commit murder.

A pelvic exam and a transvaginal sonogram performed by Connie's regular gynecologist had revealed a sixteen-weeks-size fibroid uterus, with a possible intrusion of the fibroid into the lining of her uterus (also known as the endometrial cavity).

Connie was forty-three years old, with two children, so her gynecologist thought a total hysterectomy was the answer to all her problems, especially since she did not plan to have any more children. If he also removed her ovaries, he advised, that would eliminate the possibility of ovarian cancer.

"I left my doctor's office in a fog," Connie recalled. Before that visit, her life had been good. Her marriage to Hank, an attorney, was loving, and they enjoyed their two beautiful children. The children were finally old enough to allow Connie free time for favorite activities—exercising, volunteering for charities, and her new passion, gardening. Major surgery did not fit into that relaxed and pleasant scenario.

Connie was also plagued with other symptoms. Just recently, while doing her pre-Christmas shopping, she had suffered a few "attacks," as she described them. She would suddenly become dizzy and disoriented and then overcome with a throbbing headache. After a few of these attacks, Connie realized that they always struck when she was in the perfume and cosmetics sections of department stores. Not long after, she began suffering nausea and dizziness while driving, and she realized that this happened whenever her car was near diesel-powered vehicles like buses.

Connie suspected that her problems involved something more than fibroids, so she had consulted doctors in other medical specialties. After each blood test failed to detect a problem, each doctor dismissed her symptoms. They all recommended some type of surgery to correct her fibroid condition.

The first time I met Connie and took her history, I was struck with her good health sense. She cooked organic vegetarian meals for her family. She kept few sweets in the house, and, wonder of wonders, her children followed her smart food choices.

It was easy to see why all these conventional doctors had dismissed Connie's symptoms. She appeared to be the picture of health and fitness. At five feet, four inches tall, Connie weighed a healthy 124 pounds. She exercised regularly and wisely, balancing aerobics with weight training at least five to six days a week, and always preceded and followed those workouts with stretching exercises. Connie also took time to nurture herself in other ways. She and her husband even meditated together. "Why am I being assaulted with all these symptoms?" she asked me. "I lead such a healthy life!"

"When did you last feel well?" I asked her. It is a simple question, but it can yield surprising and valuable information. Connie had no problem answering. She remembered enjoying great health until one and a half years ago. Her symptoms had surfaced in the fall following the summer she had spent putting in her new garden. Before that summer, Connie had never gardened before.

Starting in October, she recalled, she was assaulted with all sorts of mysterious ailments, including unexplained skin rashes, headaches, and sneezing fits. Her brother had always suffered from seasonal allergies, but Connie had never had that problem. A dermatologist prescribed a topical steroid cream for the rash that did get rid of it. Eventually, the headaches and other allergic symptoms also faded away, and Connie forgot about that uncomfortable autumn.

Life went back to normal until the next autumn, when all her symptoms returned, along with new complaints. Now she was suffering from abnormal periods, premenstrual symptoms, and those attacks of headaches, dizziness, and nausea. Six months later, nothing she tried helped, so Connie consulted me.

As she recounted her story, I realized that Connie had made some significant changes in her lifestyle over the past two years. Those new patterns were probably linked to her fibroid condition and other symptoms. I also suspected that the growth of her fibroids, their related symptoms, and the "attacks" stemmed from the same cause or set of causes.

At first, Connie could not think of anything new or different that had entered her life during the past two years. The only change she could pinpoint was that both her children went to sleep-away camp for the first time, leaving her with enough time to finally create the garden she had dreamed of for so long.

I asked Connie to describe how she created her garden. When she first started gardening, the earth had been overrun with insects and other pests, and the owner of her local gardening store recommended one of the strongest pesticides and insecticides available. Connie dutifully sprayed the various insects and other organisms that were destroying her new flowers, plants, and herbs, and her garden flourished. I asked Connie to fax me a list of the products she had used to kill the insects and pests. I was sure these pesticides and insecticides contained powerful xenoestrogens that had entered Connie's body through her skin, lungs, and nose, and found their way to her tissues' estrogen receptor sites. These dangerous pseudoestrogens created an estrogen-dominant state that was causing her fibroids to grow rapidly. I also suspected that these toxic foreign estrogens were the culprits behind weakened liver function, which contributed not only to her hormonal imbalance but also to her dizziness, nausea, headaches, and other symptoms. Remember, the liver is one of the body's main organs of detoxification and elimination, and it is essential in ridding the body of excess hormones. If your liver is burdened by the job of continually processing and eliminating the toxins in pesticides and insecticides, it becomes so overworked that it can no longer efficiently remove and metabolize other waste products. The other organs pitch in, attempting to pick up the slack. The skin produces rashes to help discharge wastes, and the body alerts us to the danger to the liver caused by toxic overload, by producing headaches and other symptoms. Actually, one of the doctors Connie consulted had suspected a liver problem. The conventional blood tests he had ordered came back normal, so he dismissed that possibility.

The problem with conventional liver tests is they give us information only after it is too late, when the liver is already damaged and shows signs of that dysfunction by releasing the interior of its damaged cells into the bloodstream. This is why holistic medicine uses functional liver tests, which means that these tests gauge how efficiently the liver is detoxifying toxins and handling what are called "downstream metabolites." These are fat-soluble toxins and hormones that must be changed into water-soluble substances in order to be eliminated.

All toxins and hormones are fat-soluble to begin with. This means that if they are not eliminated soon, they will be stored in the body's fat cells, where they can create harmful effects for a long time. In order to eliminate them from the body, these fat-soluble metabolites must become water-soluble metabolites so they can be excreted in urine, sweat, and stool. One of the liver's many jobs is to ready these fat-soluble substances for elimination by changing, or metabolizing, them into water-soluble products called metabolites. This conversion can occur over several stages, until the final metabolite is produced and can be efficiently excreted.

During the intermediary stages, metabolites can be even more dangerous than their initial form as toxic substances and hormones. This is particularly true if your liver is not functioning at peak. Liver function is impaired whenever it is overwhelmed by the amount of work that needs to be done or when nutritional deficiencies leave it without necessary support. Symptoms of this kind of liver toxicity include chronic fatigue, chemical sensitivities, fibromyalgia, and all types of hormonal-imbalance-linked diseases.

The tests I ordered showed that Connie suffered from compromised liver function. When she faxed me a list of the insecticides and pesticides she had used in her garden, I discovered she'd been using three different sprays. Together, they contained endosulfan, methoxychlor, and dienochlor—all potent xenoestrogens commonly found in garden sprays.

I put Connie on a powerful program to balance her hormones and detoxify and strengthen her liver, and asked her to return after six weeks.

A TYPICAL LIVER-CLEANSING PROGRAM

DIET. Liver cleansing begins with eliminating all foods that might be responsible for sensitivity reactions. Food sensitivity reactions force the liver to work hard to detoxify what the body perceives as a poison. The point is to give the liver a rest by eating hypoallergenic foods (those with low allergy potential). This usually means eliminating dairy, wheat and gluten, eggs, corn, citrus, soy, all food additives, and any food that you eat more than three to four times per week.

ULTRACLEAR PLUS. Supplement this hypoallergenic diet with a medical food called UltraClear Plus, formulated by Metagenics, that contains the nutrients the liver needs to function well. (See the resource guide.) Taking UltraClear Plus for three to six weeks allows the liver to heal and recover healthy and balanced function.

SUPPLEMENTS. Add lipotropic factors, the B vitamins choline and inositol, and sulphur-containing amino acids such as methionine to prevent and reverse fatty buildup in the liver. This helps the liver detoxify toxins much more efficiently.

HERBS. Liver antioxidants like milk thistle are helpful, as are the blood cleansers burdock, yellow dock, red clover, and artichoke to help the liver cleanse the blood efficiently. UltraClear Plus already includes lipoic acid and green tea catechins to promote healthy, balanced liver function.

CASTOR OIL PACKS. I often add castor oil packs to a liver-cleansing regimen. The packs are prepared with hexane-free castor oil (available in any health food store) and white flannel (also in health food stores). (See the resource guide for information on obtaining the packs ready-made or for purchasing the components.) You heat the castor oil to body temperature and then wet the flannel with the warmed oil. Fold the flannel so it is four layers thick. Place it over your liver. Cover the oil-soaked flannel with a plastic covering, such as a garbage bag or plastic wrap, and then lay a heating pad or other heating device over the pack. Cover with a towel to hold everything in place. Leave the pack over the liver area for at least thirty minutes. This is a great time to perform one of the meditation/visualization exercises you will learn in the following chapter. Not only does it save time, but the meditation/visualization will enhance the effect of the pack. For example, while the pack is over the liver, imagine your liver functioning in a healthy way. Your imaginary pictures do not have to be anatomically correct. Just visualize your liver any way you choose. "Seeing" it effectively getting rid of toxins and metabolizing hormones for excretion from your body can be surprisingly effective.

As soon as Connie walked in the door for her follow-up appointment, I was struck by how vibrant she appeared. Many of her symptoms—including poor sleep, fatigue, and her terrible dizziness—had improved greatly. Her one menstrual period since she had been on the program was not exactly a day at the beach, but she did notice that the bleeding was less heavy and she needed much less Motrin than usual to ease her cramps. Best of all, those awful PMS symptoms had vanished almost completely. Her emotions were much more stable, and her breasts were less tender.

We discussed adding more features to her program, but only as much as Connie felt she could take on comfortably. I do not want to increase a woman's stress load with a complicated and onerous healing regimen. The program in its entirety can appear to be daunting, especially to someone who is not accustomed to the holistic approach to health. I always tell women to start with whatever elements they feel comfortable. When they feel better, they can integrate more aspects of the program. That is also my advice to you. I once started a woman's program with Prozac only. She suffered from severe PMS, and this was the only way she could get out of bed and start her day. After she began feeling a little better, we cut back on the Prozac and gradually brought in as much of the hormone-balancing program as she could accept.

Connie was responding so well to her program that I knew the next time I saw her, in four months' time, she would look and feel even better.

The Prevalence of Toxins

One reason why protecting yourself from environmental toxins can necessitate major lifestyle changes is because they are everywhere. Studies estimate that over 100,000 man-made chemicals are currently in use in almost every industry worldwide. In 1993, for example, consumers spent $1.2 billion on 721 million pounds of dangerous chemicals, most of which are toxic xenoestrogens, though most scientists agree that these chemicals act as foreign estrogens in our bodies, with a major negative impact on human endocrine gland function.

Along with many other baby boomers. I have childhood memories of watching my dad spray our front and back yards to preserve their pristine greenness. I also remember running with my friends behind the trucks that regularly cruised our suburban neighborhoods spraying pesticides and insecticides, as part of the plan to eradicate the "evil mosquito." No one imagined at the time that those trucks carrying "helpful," disease-preventing chemicals would cause so many health problems today. Now, we are much more aware of how dangerous these chemicals really are. In 1999, New York State launched a comprehensive program to spray for mosquitoes in order to prevent a West Nile virus plague. Even though most of the spraying was done at night on a well-defined time schedule, millions of New Yorkers savvy to the chemical threat hid in their homes, windows shut, doors locked, and air conditioners turned off, in order to protect themselves from harmful chemical exposure.

Sadly, those chemicals that were sprayed so liberally in the fifties are probably still hiding out in many of our bodies. As I mentioned earlier, these fat-soluble chemicals can last for many years after they take up residence in fat cells, where they can continue exerting harmful effects long after you are first exposed. These effects can be especially harmful to the sex organs and brain, because those body parts are especially cushioned and protected by fatty tissue. Decades after DDT was banned in this country, studies show that women continue to have DDT metabolite residues in their breast milk and the fat of their breasts.

DDT and other pesticides have been banned in this country and others. A study in Israel showed that breast cancer rates decreased significantly after DDT was banned. But this dangerous chemical is still widely used among developing regions of the world. Whenever we visit these countries or eat vegetables and fruits imported from them, we risk harmful chemical exposure.

As I mentioned earlier, chemicals that disrupt normal hormone production and balance are found not only in pesticides and insecticides. They are found in our food, water, all plastics, and many other substances. The U.S. government has set legal limits for many of these harmful substances based on studies concluding that these supposedly safe amounts are not harmful. The problem is that these studies do not take into account the probability that when several of these chemicals are combined, even in legally accepted amounts, the synergy between these chemical xenoestrogens can make them much more potent than if each were acting alone. Each chemical finds its way into the body's fat cells, such as the fat cells in breast tissue, where it releases its poisons slowly and unpredictably, especially during periods of fasting and stress.

This is one reason why fasting must be done under the care of a knowledgeable health-care practitioner. When the body enters a fasting stage, it breaks down fat to help create glucose for fuel. In the process of that fat breakdown, the toxins stored in the fat are released into the blood stream. From there they travel all over the body, exerting their harmful effects. Whenever someone fasts, the liver must be supported so it can detoxify these newly released toxins more efficiently. These harmful substances actually create genetic damage to your cells by altering their DNA. By changing the

DNA, they affect not only you but potentially your future generations.

As you can see, the toxic threat to health goes beyond fibroids and other gynecological complaints. Tens of thousands of people become ill and even die each year because dangerous chemicals are still ubiquitous in our environment. You may recall a news story a few years ago involving a man in apparent good health who died suddenly, after taking a standard dose of Tylenol. An autopsy revealed that the cause of death was severe liver failure. He was a gardener who routinely used the same chemicals so many of us handle in order to keep garden pests and insects in check. It is now believed that he died because of his regular exposure to these chemicals, combined with the harmful effects of chronic nutritional deficiencies, the common deficiencies suffered by the many of us who follow the SAD program. The dose of Tylenol was simply the final straw that broke his already overburdened liver. It could not convert the Tylenol into a harmless metabolite, and the conversion process stalled halfway. The metabolism of the Tylenol did not get to the final stage of turning those Tylenol capsules into a harmless water-soluble metabolite. Instead, it never got past its intermediary stage as a killer toxin metabolite that destroyed his liver and took his life.

This story may seem like one of those bizarre and rare events that only happen to someone else. Yet similar scenarios play out all over the world, every day. People's deaths may not be as strange or dramatic, attributable to a relatively harmless, over-the-counter medication. Still, we do not really have the entire story on how some chemicals and drugs interact with the body once they have compromised liver function. Dangerous interactions between foods, drugs, and chemicals could be taking place on a daily basis. Even an herbal substance as potentially safe as Saint-John's-wort can cause bodily harm when taken alongside pharmaceutical drugs, because the liver has to metabolize and excrete both this herb and the drug via the same detoxification pathways. The successful detoxification of one substance can be severely compromised by the competing effect of the other substance.

How to Protect Yourself from the Toxic Threat

Everywhere you turn, you are surrounded by dangerous chemicals. It seems as if it is difficult, if not impossible, to escape them completely. What can you do to protect yourself?

BE AWARE. The first step is to be on the lookout for any toxins that you and your family may be exposed to.

TAKE RESPONSIBILITY. The second step is to take charge of your health by searching for the many safe and natural alternatives for common household toxins, and then make the necessary changes.

TAKE ANTI-HEAVY-METAL SUPPLEMENTS. One way to fight the toxic effects of commonly found heavy metals like aluminum is to increase in your diet the amounts of those nutrients that interfere with your body's absorption of these heavy metals and reduce their toxic effects.

Silica is a mineral that appears to reduce absorption of aluminum, which has been implicated in many disease processes, including Alzheimer's, osteoporosis, heart disease, and possibly breast cancer. Silica is often found in herbs like horsetail and in other nutrient formulas for supporting bone and collagen health.

Magnesium also seems to counter the effect of too much aluminum. This is just one more reason, among many others, to take enough of this most important mineral. An effective supplement dose is in the range of 800 to 1,200 mg a day. Remember, too much magnesium can lead to loose stools. If this occurs, simply reduce your daily intake.

Selenium and zinc are minerals that can reduce the effect in the body of other heavy toxic metals, such as cadmium and lead. A good dose of zinc is 25 mg to 50 mg a day. (Remember to take about

2 mg of copper for 30 mg of zinc.) Take 200 mcg to 400 mcg of selenium if you suspect you are contaminated with heavy metals.

Vitamin C is a natural chelating agent. "Chelate" comes from the root of the Latin word for claw. As a chelating agent, vitamin C "grabs" and binds to certain heavy metals, preventing their absorption by your body.

PROTECT YOUR WATER. Many health experts stress the importance of drinking plenty of fresh water to help your body eliminate toxins through the urine and stool. You see people carrying plastic bottles filled with various designer spring waters everywhere today. Unfortunately, these health-minded individuals often fail to realize that the soft plastic bottles containing pure water may be an added danger. My friend and colleague Dr. Alan Gaby recounts the day he decided to perform a simple experiment. He allowed spring water from a soft plastic bottle to boil off in a pan. Soon, his kitchen filled with the distinctive odor of "plastic fumes." The polychlorinated biphenyls found in soft plastic are known to be potent hormone disrupters. What we do not know for sure is whether or not we absorb these chemicals through drinking water that is bottled in soft plastic, especially if the water and container are allowed to heat up during warm summer days. Of course, we are likely to drink more water during those hot months!

One precaution you can take is to avoid leaving your water bottle in a car or any other warm place during the summer. Another good move is to invest in an insulated water bottle carrier that will keep the water temperature cool.

I also recommend installing a reputable water filtration system on your kitchen sink or keeping a supply of bottled spring water on hand. Some people arrange for a spring water company to supply them with a stand that is topped with large inverted glass bottle and a spout. The company then makes regular deliveries of new glass bottles filled with spring water. Many people think that the only safe kind of water is distilled, which means that all of the minerals are removed, along with potential impurities. My problem with distilled water is that the water loses all the helpful minerals during the distilling process. If you use distilled water, add a multimineral supplement to the water. Many liquid supplements are available to restore minerals.

REDUCE OR ELIMINATE MEAT AND DAIRY FOODS. Women with hormone imbalances and related problems such as fibroids should avoid all meat, poultry, and dairy products for at least six months while on the program so they can assess whether or not eliminating those animal products reduces fibroid growth, inflammation, and other symptoms of estrogen excess.

If you must eat meat, poultry, and dairy foods, make sure no chemical additives are present. With milk and other dairy products, avoid brands containing bovine growth hormone (BGH). We simply do not know the full range of possible health hazards associated with this and other additives, so they are best avoided. This is especially true when you are trying to heal a hormone-dependent problem by eating in a way that encourages proper hormone balance. Make sure that any meat you consume is free of hormones and antibiotics. The antibiotic residues you consume with meat help to kill off the normal balance of protective bacteria in your gut. Pathogenic or disease-causing organisms are then free to flourish and create their own toxic symptoms.

EAT DEEP-SEA COLD-WATER FISH. Deep-sea cold-water fish tend to be less contaminated with mercury and PCBs (polychlorinated biphenyls). The higher up a fish is on the food chain, the more smaller fish it has eaten, so the more likely it is to be contaminated. For instance, shark, swordfish, and marlin tend to contain higher levels of contaminants in their meat, because they have consumed smaller fish, and more harmful residues build up and concentrate in their fat. Farm-raised fish are questionable as well, because we do not know what they are fed. In order to save money, fish growers could be feeding them the same contaminated junk food that makes up the SAD nutritional program.

EAT ORGANIC FRUITS AND VEGGIES. Whenever possible, eat foods that are grown organically, with no antibiotics, pesticides, and insecticides added. This means that you need to look at food labels. Fruits and vegetables are known for their health-giving properties, but if they are not raised organically, you may be getting more than you paid for. Most fruit that is not organically produced is contaminated with insecticide and pesticide residues that can wreak havoc with your hormonal balance. Moreover, organic produce simply tastes much more delicious. After my own family began eating organic produce, it became impossible for any of us to eat a non-organic fruit or vegetable. Nonorganic tastes inferior, possibly because the "organic" label not only means less harmful additives, it means more essential minerals and other taste-giving nutrients. Another reason for the improved taste is that organic produce is allowed to grow and ripen in its own time, instead of being pumped full of gases, as are bananas, in order to force an earlier ripeness. Whether or not you do eat organic produce, always thoroughly wash your fruit and vegetables before eating.

WATCH OUT FOR GLUTEN. Remember that the gluten-containing grains—wheat, rye, oats, and barley—might be giving you a problem. Although gluten is not a toxin, now that the commercial food industry is bioengineering foods, the new gluten grains are less digestible and more allergenic. Evidence suggests that these high-gluten grains may also interfere with estrogen metabolism in the liver, thereby aggravating the state of hormonal imbalance that creates so many gynecological problems for women.

Try millet, buckwheat, and rice; they are much safer. These are also alkalinizing grains that create a less acidic environment in the body. Cancer and other abnormal growth conditions, such as fibroids, thrive in an acid environment. If you eat more acidic, less alkalinizing grains, you are creating hostile conditions that encourage abnormal growths in your body.

AVOID THE MICROWAVE. If at all possible, do not microwave foods, especially when they are wrapped in plastic. There is a good chance that plastic residues with hormone-mimicking effects could get into your food. If you do microwave, avoid this possibility by using ceramic or glass dishes. Although there is no definitive evidence that microwaving causes problems, it has been shown that it reduces the vitality of foods. I recently read about a study in which foods were photographed, using the controversial Kirlian photographic method, which is said to evaluate the energy fields that surround all living things. Food that had been microwaved appeared in the Kirlian photographs to have significantly reduced "energy" compared to foods that were not microwaved. Because of its controversial nature, I recommend microwaving as little as possible.

AVOID ALUMINUM FOIL (WITH ACIDIC FOODS). Store leftovers in another type of container, and never leave food in an opened can. Transfer it to another type container before storing.

USE NATURAL CLEANSERS AND BUG SPRAYS. Always look for natural alternatives when buying household cleansers and bug sprays. Dishwashing liquid, bathroom cleansers, laundry detergents and fabric softeners, and even safe bleach made by companies such as Ecover and Seventh Generation are all readily available at health food stores or through mail order and Internet sales companies. (See the resource guide.) These cleansing products are just as effective as their conventional, hormone-balance-disrupting equivalents. Bug sprays that use powerful and effective essential oils are just as efficient as potentially dangerous conventional insecticides, sometimes even more so.

WATCH OUT FOR NEW XENOESTROGENS. Finally, be careful of "new" and "improved" substances that could have xenoestrogen effects. I told you about the DES story in an earlier chapter. If you recall, DES, or diethylstilbestrol, was loudly touted to gynecologists by its manufacturer as a new and improved estrogen that would prevent miscarriage. The tragedy of the DES story is that not only did the drug prove ineffective against miscarriage, it also caused horrific harm. It caused such dramatic hormonal imbalances in the daughters of DES mothers that it led to a virtual plague of a previously rare vaginal cancer. DES is also responsible for numerous changes in those daughters' reproductive organs. The sons of DES mothers have suffered their own hormone-imbalance-linked diseases. Studies are now monitoring the DES daughters as they go through menopause—always a time of hormonal upheaval. In fact, researchers are also tracking the reproductive and general health of the grandchildren of DES mothers. So, the entire DES tragedy has yet to unfold. Another drug, thalidomide, made claims to be an effective sedative safe enough for pregnant women. Yet the offspring of women who took thalidomide were frequently born without arms and/or legs. That should have been a wake-up call. But we do not always learn from our mistakes.

The lesson of environmental toxins is to take responsibility for your health and to make every effort to be aware of your possible exposure to these poisons, especially since the complex workings of the female reproductive system remain, in large part, an elusive mystery. Be a lifesaver. Use caution with any new chemical products or drugs claiming profound beneficial effects. The problems they may create further down the road could be far worse than the complaints they are supposed to resolve.

9

Mental and Emotional Fibroid Healing

You have learned that the stress of unresolved issues and emotions can help set you up for hormonal imbalance and fibroids. The muscular effort of trying to suppress these painful memories and emotions can create, over time, a tight band of chronically contracted muscles and fascial tissue (the tissue covering and supporting muscle groups). This tight band restricts free movement of the pelvis and "freezes" the lower abdomen. Circulation, breathing, and energy become limited, leading to low vitality and, among other health problems, gynecological disorders.

From the eastern medical perspective, this muscular "armor" creates energy stagnation that is a prelude to tumor formation. Think of energy as water. When nothing obstructs it, water flows freely and stays pure and healthy. As soon as water flow is dammed up, though, waste and sludge build. If that water is allowed to remain stagnant, the muck increases and can even become semisolid. Little moves in this thick accumulation of debris. According to eastern thought, that same phenomenon occurs in the body wherever the life force is blocked and allowed to stagnate.

◆ Diane's Story

Diane was a registered nurse who performed her duties with great efficiency. She also took excellent care of her own health, so she was mystified by the recent appearance of serious gynecological problems. Her periods had become heavy and painful. Sex was difficult because of a constant sense of abdominal pressure, and she had even started to leak urine whenever she jumped or engaged in any other strenuous activity. Diane was diagnosed with subserous and intramural fibroids and told to get a hysterectomy. She came to my office for a second opinion.

During our interview, Diane mentioned the abuse she had suffered as a child at the hands of a violent and alcoholic stepfather. Diane had never considered that her fibroids and other gynecological problems could be related to this unresolved issue, but she was willing to explore a possible connection.

I recommended a brief course of psychotherapy to help her express feelings about her unhappy experiences and release emotions that she had kept bottled up for many years. I encouraged her to embark on daily meditation-visualization sessions to help her further in achieving closure with the past. Diane also began practicing other body-mind techniques to soften the protective armor of chronically tight bands of muscle and fascia around her lower torso. That muscular armor had helped her repress painful emotions from conscious awareness, but, at the same time, it was blocking energy from her pelvic area and aggravating her gynecological symptoms.

The chronically tight muscles that protect us from painful emotions lower vitality, in part, because they impede full breathing. With the breath unable to flow freely in and out of the lower abdominal area, energy stagnation sets in. Another way in which suppressed emotions and memories have a negative effect on health is by breeding negative and self-limiting thoughts. No matter how we struggle to hold it down, no disturbing emotion or memory can ever be totally blocked. That pain will express itself however it can, often by creating a negative habit of thinking. All this makes you vulnerable to many different health problems, including fibroid tumors.

Reichian and Bioenergetic Theory and Practice

Repressed emotions can be triggered by an early trauma that induced terror, grief, or sexual shame. Those emotions and memories do not just go away. They are simply held in check by the viselike grip of rigid muscles and fascial supporting tissue. Imagine how much vitality you lose after years, even decades, because you have been expending so much energy on the struggle to keep those suppressed memories and emotions in check.

When those rigid tissues are released through special breathing and physical exercises, their accompanying emotions are also freed and your energy is liberated.

Reichian therapy (developed by Wilhelm Reich) and its offshoots—bioenergetics and other body-mind therapies practiced today—developed these exercises to liberate emotions and the energy they hold from the muscular-fascial defense system. When those muscular contractions are released (especially those constricting pelvic and abdominal movement), you are able tolerate a far deeper level of energy in your torso, and your body is better able to make its own corrections to restore balance and health.

To continue our water analogy, visualize what happens to water that has been dammed up when the obstruction is finally removed. The water begins to flow freely once again, clearing away the accumulated debris and waste in its path.

Eastern healers describe the same relationship between emotions and health in their own unique terms. They link gynecological dysfunction, including fibroids, to disturbances in what is known as second chakra energy. Each chakra is roughly analogous to the endocrine glands that supply the body with hormones, and also comparable to each of the nerve plexuses that run along the spinal column. Each chakra also represents a specific energy that relates to a different facet of our collective human experience. The second chakra corresponds to the second nerve plexus from the bottom of the spine. The human experience, issues, and emotions associated with the second chakra include our relationships to money, power, people, jobs, creativity, and sexuality. In other words, second chakra issues relate to those elements of your life that are in your way or those elements you want and/or need to create in your life but, for some reason, cannot. The second chakra also relates to issues of abuse. In fact, most experts are convinced of the connection between sexual abuse and the development of fibroids. A recent study that was reported in a medical-peer-review journal identified an association between chronic pelvic pain and unresolved issues related to past sexual abuse. Childhood abuse does not have to be sexual. Emotional abuse and other types of physical abuse can also lead to energy stagnation in the pelvic area, the part of the body governed by the second chakra. I have noted that many of my patients who suffer from fibroids and other chronic gynecological ailments are also plagued with second-chakra-related emotional issues.

The insights gained by psychotherapy and the energy liberation promised by body-mind release techniques are not the only way to address this problem of energy stagnation. You can also use other techniques to help you achieve the focus and calm that improves health and better equips you to heal your fibroid condition. These simple and enjoyable practices allow buried issues and emotions to emerge gradually. As they rise into your conscious awareness, they often lose their power to restrict your energy and health. I have observed such eastern healing techniques as acupuncture, acupressure, and chi gong address the problem of energy stagnation effectively by promoting unimpeded free flow of the life-force energy that maintains optimal health.

Relaxation, Meditation, and Visualization

Relaxation and visualization techniques are among the most powerful ways to counter self-limiting thoughts that may be blocking your healing. If you are worried that you lack enough imagination or ability to practice visualization techniques, a simple exercise described later in this chapter will put you in touch with your natural facility.

One simple and effective strategy for correcting energy disturbances is to cultivate a daily meditation and visualization practice. There are two authors who have been particularly successful in helping people learn how to use imagery for healing. Gerald Epstein, who has a private practice in New York City and has written extensively on the subject, and O. Carl Simonton, who came out in the seventies with the groundbreaking book on the subject, *Getting Well Again*. Though Simonton's book concerns the use of visualization techniques for healing cancer, his strategies can easily be applied to any condition.

Meditation

Transcendental meditation has been proven to help relieve a host of health complaints. So have other simple meditation techniques in which people focus on the rhythm of their inhalations and exhalations or on a single sound. The purpose of these exercises is to cultivate a nonreactive, in-the-moment state of mind that encourages focused energy and promotes the clarity and calm that helps release and direct healing energy.

In *Why People Don't Heal*, Carolyn Myss explains what happens to us when we expend energy on worrying about possible scenarios that have not even occurred or fretting about events that already took place. We leave little energy for the present moment and we cannot focus on effecting a successful healing. All meditation practices help us train as much of our energy as possible on the moment, so we are able to create whatever elements or changes we want in our lives. It has been said many times and in many ways that the past is gone and the future has not yet arrived, so the only effective place to put your effort to work is the present.

Meditation can also involve physical elements. The breath work and physical "flow" activity included in yoga, Taoist exercises, tai chi, chi gong, and other Eastern disciplines increase awareness of the harmony between body and mind, reduce stress, and promote physical and mental flexibility. Actually, any activity that allows you to "get into the flow," where time seems to stand still, becomes an effective meditation tool and stress reducer. These activities cover a wide spectrum—from the highly ritualized Japanese tea ceremony to such common, everyday activities as dusting furniture. My wife, Priscilla, does all the cooking in our home, and my job is to clean up after meals. I have transformed dishwashing from an onerous task to a meditation activity that allows me to stay in the moment, calm my mind, reduce stress on my adrenal glands, and reduce the stress from my day in the office. All this promotes hormonal balance, healing, and good health.

In *Flow: The Psychology of Optimal Experience,* Mihaly Csikszentmihalyi describes this state in which the individual is totally absorbed in the experience of the moment, without fretting about the past or worrying about the future. During these experiences, time appears to stand still and healing increases. As a young boy, my eldest son, Adam, played soccer. Whenever he would recount an exceptionally good play he'd made, he'd tell me that, at that moment, nothing other than the game was in his mind and "time seemed to stand still." That sense of timelessness and complete engagement in the present is exactly what a regular meditation practice encourages. When we are fully in the flow, we are the most effective in cocreating our lives.

Visualizations

Visualizations are simple but powerful meditative techniques that also should be part of any effective and lasting healing program. Instead of just focusing on a sound or your breath, you use a meditative state of mind to imagine your healing, exactly the way you want it. First, you place yourself in a focused and calm meditative state.

Then, you invest the power of all your belief in a detailed scenario that portrays the ideal outcome of a particular situation. Most of my patients who are struggling with fibroids imagine "seeing," in their mind's eye, their fibroids shrinking in a healthy, balanced pelvic area. When you perform these visualizations, use as many senses as you can. In addition to "seeing" what is going on in your pelvis, you might also "smell" pleasant odors, feel the textures of the fibroid, feel your uterus free of fibroids, and "hear" healthy blood flowing freely to nourish the area. The more senses used, the more powerful the visualization.

Regular journal writing can make you more aware of any feelings, thoughts, or memories that come up during your meditation and visualization sessions. Some patients also make drawings or paintings of their uterus and fibroids and what they "see" during their visualization sessions. I have also recommended to some patients who find it difficult to do visualizations that they sculpt their uterus and its fibroids in clay or another pliable material. In this way, they are better able to understand and visualize what is going on in that area. Once they can do that, they can more easily move on to visualizing the changes they want to see take place. These practices also help to get that stored energy out of the pelvis and into the light, where it can be worked on.

Guided Visualization Exercise

Try this simple exercise. Close your eyes, and try to make your mind an absolute blank for a few moments.

What is happening? Does your attention keep wandering to the sounds of traffic outside, the wind rustling in the trees, the list of chores you must complete today, that argument you had with your friend last week, the rumbling in your tummy telling you it is time for lunch, or the little voice in your head that urges, "Hey! Let's get some pizza"?

If all this interference is sullying that perfect blankness you are aiming for, don't worry. You're normal. Only seasoned meditators can observe that passing parade of mind talk with distance and objectivity. That takes a lot of practice. In fact, it is the reason why meditation *practice* is called practice—because you are always learning. Keep in mind that whatever you are doing is perfect for where you are right now. As you continue to practice, you will find it easier to focus and resist distractions. Even though these distractions may always enter your consciousness, you will learn to view them with objectivity and not get stuck on them. The practice of meditation does not mean keeping all extraneous thoughts out of your mind, but it does mean that you no longer expend energy on them.

So guided visualizations differ from meditation because your mind is given a script to follow, making it more difficult for your mind to wander wherever it will. The script is tailored specifically to you, written with the goal of liberating yourself from any thoughts and belief systems that are inhibiting your healing and compromising your health.

If you can visualize in precise detail all the changes you want in your life—painting a vivid mental picture of your life just as you wish it to be—almost by magic, your reality will begin conforming to that image. Barbara Levine, a writer on this subject, titled her book *Your Body Believes Every Word You Say.* Levine describes the connection between what the mind has to say and the body's obedient response. By observing and editing the messages of your mind, you can have a direct and positive effect on your body's healing.

RELAXATION TECHNIQUES

Before you can reap the benefits of guided visualizations, you must first learn to relax as completely as possible. You can accept and incorporate alternative beliefs much more easily when you are relaxed. You are more open for "reprogramming," for taking in suggestions on new patterns of thought and behavior regarding your health that will eventually replace the negative thoughts and behaviors.

Relaxation training begins with focusing on the breath and muscle tension, and then progresses to allowing thoughts to drift into and out of the mind, rather than hanging on to any worrisome thoughts that are already there. In this relaxed state, you can distance yourself from negative thoughts and emotions about your condition and make room for the positive images of your guided visualization. At the same time, releasing any tension you feel in your body goes a long way toward deepening the "relaxation response," a term coined by Dr. Herbert Benson to describe the profound meditative state that can be achieved with progressive relaxation of the body.

The ideal mind state for a guided visualization is one of relaxed attention: You are alert and concentrated on what is happening inside you. At the same time, though, you are uninvolved with what may be happening on the outside.

It is important to understand that this kind of relaxation means time alone in a quiet environment where you will not be disturbed, even by the telephone or doorbell. It does not mean lying on the sofa with your feet up, mesmerized by the boob tube.

During deep relaxation, refrain from any other activity.

Research has shown that for deep relaxation to be effective, you must have at least one period of relaxation daily, lasting a minimum of fifteen to twenty minutes. This may be too much of a challenge for beginners, so it is all right to start with sessions lasting only five to ten minutes. Remember Delores, the dutiful wife and mother who thought that taking any time for her own needs was selfish? Her meditation practice began with lying in bed while taking her basal body temperature for seven minutes every morning for a few days. A venerable Chinese saying reminds us that the longest journey starts with one step. The same is true about relaxation training, meditation, visualizations, and any other aspect of a healing program. The most important step is the first.

Relaxation training begins by focusing on breathing and muscle relaxation. It does not matter which relaxation technique you use.

What does matter is that you have a consistent and deep experience of relaxation. In such a state, thoughts occur less frequently and do not become fixations. Your breathing becomes slow and steady, and your muscles feel deeply relaxed. This state might be characterized by a heavy, weighty sense of your body, or the opposite, a light, floating sensation. People often report feeling quiet, focused, and passive. All these sensations are usually indications that you are deeply relaxed. Thoughts will enter your mind, but you will not dwell on them. The mind becomes like a movie screen with images moving across it. Each picture-thought is observed as it moves into the frame of your consciousness. Then, it is allowed to move just as easily out of the frame of your consciousness. You do not freeze any frames, that is, you do not hang on to any thought.

CONTRACTION-RELEASE

One of the most common methods of relaxation is based on the principle of "contraction-release" in which you tense and then relax successive muscle groups of your body. When tensing a group of muscles, hold them as tightly as possible, then let go and relax completely. Best results are gained through regular practice. You can even tape-record these instructions, which lends an added self-help element because your own voice is helping you through the exercise. Another option is to play soothing music in the background.

- Arrange your body in a comfortable position. Lying on your back on the floor or in bed is preferable, but you may sit in a chair if you wish. Uncross your legs and extend your arms along your sides, palms facing up.
- Take three long, full inhalations into your lower abdomen. You should actually feel the breath traveling down into the pelvis, where it fills that area completely. Exhale completely each time. Feel your body let go of tension with each exhalation and sink more and more deeply into the floor or mattress.
- Clench your right fist and hold the tension there, tighter

and tighter. Study the tension in your right fist as you keep the rest of your body relaxed. Then drop the tension and allow a sensation of relaxation to flow in. Observe the difference between relaxation and tension as a pleasant, heavy feeling floods your hand—into your palm, into each finger.

• Now, clench your left fist, then release the tension in the same manner as above.

• Clench both fists and straighten both arms, tensing the muscles. Hold the tension. Observe the tension. Now release the tension in both arms and let them drop to your sides. Observe the warm, heavy feeling of relaxation flowing into your arms, down the elbows, through the wrists, into the palms. Feel yourself letting go, relaxing. Take a long, deep breath. Exhale slowly, becoming even more relaxed and centered in your body.

• Take another long, deep breath, filling your lungs. Hold the air in your chest, observing the tension created. Now exhale slowly, observing the walls of your chest loosen as the air is pushed out. Continue relaxing and breathing freely and gently. With each exhalation feel yourself sinking deeper and deeper into the floor or the mattress.

• Tighten your abdominal muscles by pushing them up and out as far as they can go. Hold the tension there and study it. Release the abdominal muscles and allow the feeling of relaxation to flow into each muscle. Continue breathing freely and easily. On each exhalation, notice the pleasant sensation of relaxation spreading throughout your body.

• Tense your buttocks and thighs by pressing down as hard as you can and clenching your buttocks muscles together. Hold the tension and study it. Release and allow a deep, soothing feeling of relaxation to flow in.

• Tense your lower legs by pressing both feet down as hard as you can and pinching your calf muscles together. Hold the tension and study it. Release and allow a deep, soothing feeling of relaxation to flow in. Breathe in and out easily and allow relaxation to flow throughout your body.

- Tense your back and shoulders by pinching your shoulders together and arching your back off the floor. Hold the tension and let go, allowing your back to drop gently down to the floor. Feel the relaxation spread.

- Roll your head back and forth very gently from side to side, releasing the muscles in the back of your neck.

- Tense your facial muscles by sticking out your tongue as far as it will go, closing your eyes tightly, and wrinkling up your forehead. Hold the tension, then release, allowing warm relaxation to flow through the scalp, forehead, eyelids, cheeks, jaw, even your tongue.

- Now, allow your body to experience heaviness, as if it is boneless and only the floor is keeping you from sinking. You may, at this time, make a mental inventory of the parts of your body you have contracted and released, telling yourself as you go through your body that each part is heavy, warm, and relaxed.

- When you are ready to enter the waking state, begin by gently wriggling toes and fingers, gradually moving into whatever larger stretches your body wants.

- Roll to one side in a fetal position, place one palm on the floor, and push off, lifting your body comfortably and easily into a sitting position.

BELLY BREATHING

This simple form of relaxation demonstrates the relaxing effects of the diaphragmatic, or belly, breath that is similar to the Basic Eastern Breath you learned in Chapter 7.

- First, inhale quickly, expanding your chest cavity as much as you can and letting your shoulders rise. Exhale. Repeat this for three to five cycles. You may not even reach three cycles before you begin to feel tense, anxious, and even a bit lightheaded.

- Now contrast those sensations with the relaxed calm you

238 ✦ HEALING FIBROIDS

experience with belly breathing. Place both hands on your lower belly, just below the belly button. Take several slow, deep inhalations so that your belly pushes out against your hands. Feel your inhalations actually pushing your hands off your belly. Do this for as long as you like. Directing your inhalations into your belly and allowing your exhalations to be long and easy makes for a profoundly relaxing meditation session. Relax your entire body as completely as you can. Breathe in through your nose in a natural, easy way.

• Exhale slowly through your mouth, emptying the belly, letting your jaw relax and drop. Make each exhalation last as long as possible, but do not hold the breath between inhalations and exhalations.

• Each time you inhale, feel the breath travel farther downward, all the way to the diaphragm, where it loosens those muscles, then all the way to the bottom of your belly, where it loosens the pelvic girdle. Remember to allow your belly to expand gently as you take in each breath. Keep your shoulders and chest relaxed and still. As you allow the diaphragm to descend with each inhalation, feel the energy of that inhalation massage the abdominal and pelvic organs. Try this next time you have eaten too much good food and feel as if you are about to burst. Deep belly breathing can relieve abdominal discomfort with its gentle intestinal massage.

Once you have learned to put yourself in a state of deep relaxation at will, you can simply give yourself an image or word, such as "relax" or "breathe" to trigger that state. At that point, you will be equipped to become a masterful creator of guided visualizations that can greatly enhance your health. I often use the phrase "right now" to get myself into a relaxed state. I say "right" to myself on the in breath, and "now" on the out breath. This simple technique helps me remain focused on the present moment.

Start with the following simple exercises that combine relaxation with guided visualization.

Relaxation/Visualization Exercises

The following visualizations help relax, cleanse, and heal—physically and mentally.

ENERGY FLOW VISUALIZATION

This visualization promotes the free flow of life-force energy into, through, and out of your body, leaving you feeling more vibrant and energized.

- Begin, as always, by relaxing your body and breathing deeply and naturally. Do not begin until you feel relaxed.
- Focus your vision inward. Each time you inhale, see a golden, sunlit energy streaming through your body, warming you, revitalizing, energizing, and cleansing.
- Inhale a wave of healing energy that moves up the front of your body. The wave begins at your toes, and, with each inhalation, moves farther toward the top of your head.
- When the energy reaches the crown of your head, inhale several more times, each time bringing the wave of light from your toes to your head in a single breath.
- With each exhalation, see this brilliant sun energy move down the back of your body, out the backs of your heels and into the ground.
- Now, inhale and circle your entire body with the golden energy. Do this several times.
- As you watch the energy circle through your body, notice areas of tension and blockage. Direct the golden light with your breath and mind-force into those areas to unblock, release, and soothe them.
- See the golden energy penetrating every cell and fiber, massaging every part of your inner body with warming, purifying radiance. Know that as the light enters your body through your toes, it brings cleansing and purifying energy. As it leaves your body through the backs of your heels, it takes away any im-

purities, tensions, negative thoughts, and worries. Wherever you sense disharmony, bring in this healing golden energy. See the golden energy surround and pervade every cell in the area. This is the energy that will help heal your condition, whether it is fibroids or any other physical problem.

• When you feel completely relaxed, purified, and revitalized, open your eyes and gently return to the present physical reality.

Body Scan Meditation

This powerful healing meditation technique was developed by Jon Kabat-Zinn, of the University of Massachusetts Stress Reduction Clinic. It involves moving your awareness to various parts of your body to help you tune in to your body and evaluate where you need attention and healing. In my medical practice, I teach my patients to do body scans to help them increase awareness and sensitivity to their pelvic organs. First, I do an ultrasound exam to show them the condition of the uterus and ovaries. Then I explain how to do the body scan.

This process returns to us an element of control by encouraging awareness, responsibility, and self-determination. I do the body scan technique myself most mornings, before I get out of bed. It takes twenty to thirty minutes and is extremely relaxing. Body scan meditation is a key part of my own self-nurturing, and it allows me to interact with the world in a holistic way. As you remember, giving your adrenal glands sufficient rest is essential to maintaining ideal hormone balance. The technique is simple:

• Begin with several deep and even belly breaths. Feel yourself become more relaxed and your body grow heavier with each exhalation.
• Turn your awareness to your feet, allowing yourself to feel

any and all sensations in that part of your body. Feel the pressure of the floor or mattress against your heels. A blanket may be lying on top of your toes. Feel that. You might sense some pain or ache in a bunion or ingrown toenail. Move your attention to the sensation and direct your breath more fully into the feeling. Be aware of any thoughts that arise as you move more deeply into the pain or sensation. Do not attempt to push these thoughts away. The thoughts may be messages from the condition, telling you what needs to be dealt with in order for healing to occur. If you can write down these thoughts after you complete the body scan, you will be better able to understand the "message" of malady, whether it is a bunion, a backache, or a fibroid uterus. Are there any colors? Any smells? Do you suddenly find yourself thinking about a particular incident in your past that you never connected before to this feeling or to your fibroid condition? These thought-messages could lead you to the key issues at the root of your malady.

• Next, direct your breath into your feet, where it brings energy and healing light.

• Repeat the above steps with each part of your body, moving up to legs, knees, thighs, pelvis, and buttocks—until you reach your head.

• At this point, allow the breath to come in through the top of the head and travel down your body to your feet.

After only a brief period of regular body scanning, you will sense a certain rhythm between your body and your breath, as you inhale and exhale out of various parts.

Whenever you feel a sensitive area at any point during your body scan, move your consciousness into that place, along with healing energy. At the same time, you can spontaneously create a healing image. I strongly believe that we are all capable of healing ourselves in this way. Perform this simple exercise regularly and you will be surprised by its effectiveness.

PURIFYING FIRE VISUALIZATION

This is an effective exercise in which your mind power and breath energize and cleanse your body of toxins, muscular tensions, and negative beliefs about your ability to heal.

- Lie on your back, legs extended, feet about hip-width apart, arms slightly away from your sides.
- Focus your attention on the crown, or top, of your head.
- Now, shift your focus to the soles of your feet.
- Become aware of the space between the crown of your head and the soles of your feet. See that space as an empty container waiting to be filled and cleansed with the purifying energy of your breath.
- Now inhale deeply through the bottoms of your feet as you visualize pure, white, sparkling life-force energy moving up and filling the container of your body.
- As the purifying light passes through your body, see all physical impurities and tensions, all fatigue, all negative beliefs and emotions, as dried autumn leaves. The light is gathering up these leaves and carrying them upward.
- As you exhale slowly and evenly, see the dried leaves exiting through your mouth and nostrils and combusting into brilliant flames that incinerate them completely.
- Keep inhaling the leaves upward and exhaling them into a fiery nothingness. Hear the leaves crackle as they burn up and disintegrate into ash. Smell them burn. Do this until no more leaves are left, and you are full of sparkling pure light.

TANTRIC COLOR MEDITATION

Tantric practitioners and increasing numbers of Westerners know that color exerts a powerful effect on our minds and bodies. Scientists have even proven that violet increases the activity of the female hormone glands. This exercise uses color to increase your energy and gynecological health.

- Sit in a comfortable cross-legged position or in a straight-back chair, making sure your spine is straight and shoulders relaxed.
- Close your eyes and visualize radiant colors—brilliant rays of red, orange, yellow, green, blue, indigo, and violet—pouring over you in a warm, life-giving flood. Feel each color's luminous energy penetrate each cell.
- Relax, letting your entire body go limp for a few moments.
- Sit upright again and exhale all the air from the lungs, forcing it out by contracting your abdomen.
- Inhale slowly, expanding your abdomen. Hold your breath for the count of seven, as you visualize the color violet. See the rays of violet flowing over your lower abdomen and genital area, then see violet covering the back of your head.
- Repeat this process three times.

Tantrics advise practicing this color meditation in front of an open window or outdoors, in sunlight.

Creating Your Own Guided Visualization Scenarios

Your own guided visualizations are like choreographed daydreams, a script you write, then rehearse until it is ready to perform and become your day-to-day reality. Going over that scripted visualization is like focusing your inner projector, or inner eye, on the inner movie screen of your mind.

There is no right or wrong way to do a guided visualization; all that counts is that it produces the results you are after. The degree to which that visualization becomes part of your actual life experience depends, though, on how carefully you create the scenario and how much belief you invest in it.

First, you need to decide precisely and in minute detail what you really want. You may want to write your script—either in your head or on paper—then see how it looks on your inner movie screen, editing it and making additions as it plays out.

Remember to beware of answered prayers. Make sure that these images reflect the *exact* changes that will actually give you the outcome you desire. We all ask for various items and outcomes when praying, but sometimes the most effective prayer is the one that asks for whatever outcome will bring us the most good. In this way, we trust the wisdom of the universe without presuming that we know better. Whenever I am about to do a surgical procedure, I practice a visualization exercise. I see in my mind's eye the entire procedure carried out without any complications. I visualize the patient having a swift and uncomplicated postoperative course. Most important, I feel myself connect with the wisdom and energy of the universe. I ask for guidance and strength so that I can perform at my best. I also ask the patient to do a visualization that I believe helps prevent excessive bleeding and any other negative effects from the procedure. I ask my patients to see the blood vessels that lead into the area as pipes with turn-off valves. I tell them to practice turning off all the valves in their minds, until there is no blood flow into the area being operated on. They practice turning the valves on and off until they can do it easily. I then advise them—tongue in cheek—that they had better not forget to turn the valves back on during their practice, because I wouldn't want anyone to suffer from psychically induced gangrene. Then, when they are about to be anesthetized, they do the same visualization and leave the values turned off.

TIPS FOR CREATING AN EFFECTIVE VISUALIZATION

• Make the images of your visualization as clear, specific, and lifelike as possible. Do not worry about being anatomically correct about whatever you visualize. Some women visualize sharks and pac-men gobbling up their fibroids. Others see the herbs they are taking dissolving the fibroid. There is no single correct way. Whatever feels comfortable and right will be effective for you.

• Your visualization does not have to conform to the constraints of ordinary reality in any way. It can follow dream logic, where anything goes. You can fly or see energy build in your body as vivid colors, textures, and shapes.

• Focus not just on your goal but on how you will get there, the process. See the entire experience: You are eating well, exercising regularly, taking healing herbs and supplements. You begin feeling more energetic, less troubled by pain and other symptoms. See your fibroids shrink smaller and smaller until they disappear. Do not leave out a single detail, and take your time in visualizing each moment of your healing. For example, if a pregnancy is your ultimate goal, see the baby in the uterus. Visualize the baby's birth. See, feel, hear, and smell the baby. If you have a dedicated partner, ask him to do this meditation with you. Hold hands as both of you "see" the same things happening, to deepen and intensify the visualization's effectiveness.

I will never forget my experience with a patient I will call Trudy. Many years ago, when she was about twenty-three years old and childless, Trudy was under my care in the hospital for a severe pelvic abscess. She had suffered several bouts of pelvic inflammatory disease that stemmed from an IUD inserted by another gynecologist a few years earlier. Trudy had been getting two intravenous antibiotics for a few days. On Sunday morning, she showed signs that her abscess was leaking. A leaking abscess usually requires surgery, and surgery in Trudy's case would probably have meant a total hysterectomy. At this time, I was meditating regularly on my own but had not yet incorporated it into my practice. I decided to try guided imagery as part of Trudy's treatment. She had a devoted husband and an exceptionally close relationship with her father. It was not unusual for both men to spend most of the day with her in the hospital. I wanted to use the closeness of these relationships to enhance the visualization. So, after I added a third antibiotic to the intravenous mixture, I explained to Trudy, her father, and her husband how the antibiotics were working to cure her infection.

I asked them to hold hands and visualize together how the medicines were working in her body and to "see" the infection disappearing. Then I went home and did my own visualization of Trudy's healing. Of course, all that afternoon I was waiting for the phone call that would send me rushing back to the hospital to perform emergency surgery. That call never came. The next day Trudy was significantly improved, and she left the hospital with all her organs intact. Unfortunately, Trudy moved out of the area, so I never found out if she was ever able to get pregnant, but the incident impressed me with how visualizations can affect healing.

• Whatever you are visualizing must be seen as happening now. Do not see yourself in optimal health sometime in the future. Stay in the present moment, in the eternal now. This is similar to the concept behind affirmations. Instead of saying, "My fibroids will be gone by my next checkup," affirm that "My fibroids are gone and my pelvis is whole and healthy right now."

• Involve as many of your senses as possible to make your scenario even more real. Feel, hear, taste, even smell, whatever you are seeing.

• As these images of your healing pass by, sense how each one makes you feel. Do you really want that? Is something else missing from your healing experience that needs to be there before you can fulfill that ultimate goal?

• Be aware of all the feelings that arise as you spin out this scenario. Do you feel a yearning for something elusive, an excited anticipation, or the calm sense of completion that comes with accomplishing a goal? Whatever feelings or sensations come up, accept them and experience them fully. They will bring you closer to fulfilling your goal.

• Whenever a particularly appealing image flashes on your inner screen, freeze the frame. Savor that image for a few moments, as you tell yourself it is already yours.

• Affirm aloud that you deserve the very best life has to offer, especially a healthy, fulfilling life. I like to use this powerful affirmation: "Prosperity and comfort surround me, and I am blessed with abundant health."

• Be patient. It may take several tries to get going, and results may not show right away, but they will come. You need time and patience, and remember to welcome any persistent doubts and blocks because they tell you where you need to go next. Thomas Edison once said, "Many failures in life are people who did not know how close they were to success when they gave up."

• Do not forget to include in your visualization whatever you think is missing from your life that will help you effect a complete healing. Focus on the vision of yourself in perfect health, free of fibroids.

• After you have visualized all the details of your healing, *then* end your imaginary scenario with an image of you enjoying life and perfect health. Finally, I like to end my visualization session with the feeling that my personal boundaries have dissolved so I can experience my profound connection with the energy of the universe. To me, there is nothing more restorative.

• Do not worry about whether or not your goal is realistic. The mind can work miracles. Have faith and apply a little effort, time, and patience.

How to Deal with Negative Thoughts

If you find you are unable to visualize a particular feeling or experience, explore that block and try to discover why you are avoiding or protecting yourself from that particular experience. Explore any strong negative feelings associated with that block—fear, anger, anxiety, or irritation. Do not try to suppress them. Do this by asking yourself why you are feeling this way. This is how you will discover what has been blocking your authentic health all along.

Two common negating thoughts are: "I'll never be able to do that!" and "I'm too sick to heal myself." Do they sound familiar?

Once you uncover your negative thoughts and beliefs, you will realize that you were already playing out a visualization without even knowing it: a negative, nonstop scenario about your health that was feeding you an endless loop of defeating suggestions. Do not be afraid to let *that* movie play out in your mind a few more times, until you can see it clearly for the lie that it is.

Give yourself the same sound counsel you would give a friend. Switch from being your own worst enemy to becoming your own best friend. Challenge the validity of your negative thoughts and the feelings they create. Get professional help if necessary to overcome these obstacles to your healing and replace these thoughts with more positive beliefs that will create a fulfilling reality.

Remember, you cannot enjoy a truly complete healing without first cleansing the mind of worn-out, unfulfilling, and—even worse—destructive patterns.

Your will and energy are the engine of your visualization, so be open to doing whatever it takes to make real whatever you have imagined. Even if you do not entirely believe that a guided visualization can change your fibroid condition, *pretend* that it will. The power of pretending cannot be undervalued.

Try this the next time you feel sad, angry, or worried. First, see in your mind's eye your face as it is now, wearing a frown or a scowl. Do you like this look? Do you feel entitled to that face because of the woes that have befallen you? Maybe so.

Now, picture your face wearing a smile. Since you are such a good visualizer by now, it should not be difficult. You may not achieve an ear-to-ear grin, but begin to reverse the direction of that frown or scowl, and you will be amazed at how much better you will feel. That is the power of the body-mind/mind-body connection. Over time, pretending develops into a habit of positive thinking and shifts the creations of your imagination into the realm of genuine possibility.

After you become accomplished in guided visualization techniques, all you will have to do is give yourself a preset signal to relax, then turn your mind briefly to an image or images of what you want in your life, and you will create it. To me, that is what is meant when it was written that we were created in God's image—being the cocreators of our lives.

Develop Your Imaginative Powers

You may still be saying to yourself, "Sure, that's fine for some, but I have no imagination and my mind constantly wanders. I can't do this!"

Recent research on guided imagery does indicate that about 10 percent of people are particularly imaginative, what researchers call "high absorbers." Any sensory stimulation—a piece of music, a beautiful panorama in nature, a whiff of an appealing scent—and their imaginations are so stimulated that they are swept away by a flood of fantasy that packs all the impact of reality.

A high absorber could probably enjoy perfect health simply by conjuring it up in her mind.

The good news is that with practice, you could do that, too. We all have a degree of imaginative power, and it can be developed fairly easily.

In fact, if you are practicing any of the breathing, relaxation, and guided imagery exercises you have read about so far, you have already begun to stimulate and enhance your imaginative faculties.

Here is a helpful exercise to develop your imagination.

Read each of the items on the list that follows. See each one as an image in your mind. Take your time. Do this every day for a week. Then, one by one, bring in each of your other senses: smell, taste, touch, hearing. Practice each sense daily for a few days. Stop for a week or so. Then, go over the list, first seeing images of the words, then smelling, tasting, touching, and hearing them.

Items

    Your father's face

    Your unmade bed

A barking dog
A purring kitten
A speeding motorcycle
A stoplight
Your favorite chair or sofa
Ocean waves lapping at the shore
Your best friend
Soft fur
A skin rash
Your morning shower
You jumping as high as you can
Brushing your teeth
You eating chocolate
Coffee percolating (or your favorite tea brewing)
Your favorite flower
A child playing
An intense sexual experience

It will not be long before you will notice how much easier it is for each item to set off a rush of vivid images, sounds, smells, tastes, and feelings. You will soon realize that you do have a good imagination, after all.

Finally, it is most helpful if you can view your fibroid condition as a valuable life lesson that is calling on you to become your own healer and to create a more meaningful and fulfilling life. Your healing may be connected to such essential questions as "What is the energy of this part of my body—the pelvis and sex organs and glands—all about?" "What does this energy mean in terms of my own emotions and drives?" "How does this energy relate to my own fibroid condition?" "What is the message of this fibroid?"

Once you have embarked on the journey to find answers, you will realize that you have responded to the challenge of a difficult health problem by becoming a stronger, more self-aware and responsible person.

10

Putting Your Own Healing Program Together

Everything you've read so far about how to heal fibroids reflects the four principles of holistic medicine that I told you about in Chapter 3. These four principles, plus other strategies that I will describe in this chapter, will help you use the information you have gained from this book to take charge of your own healing.

- Address the whole person—body, mind, and spirit—by integrating conventional and alternative therapies.

You have learned how to balance your physical health. This includes not only eating the right foods so that your body receives the nutrients it needs to perform at peak balance and energy, but also minding *how* you eat (which even includes with *whom* you eat!). Also included in the program's attention to your physical health is improving the quality of your digestion and elimination, to make your body an environment in which fibroids do not thrive. You have also learned how environmental toxins called xenoestrogens can aggravate the condition of estrogen dominance that influences fibroid growth and how removing these toxins, through avoidance and/or detoxification, can reduce fibroid growth and symptoms of estrogen dominance.

- Balance attention to relieving symptoms with eliminating their root causes.

We have covered a wide range of possible causes for a fibroid condition, many of which do not fall into the usual concerns of a gynecological practice, because each bodily function is intricately related to all the others. As you learned, possible contributing causes for fibroids include problems with intestinal and liver function, exposure to xenoestrogens, nutritional deficiencies, hormone imbalances, and emotional issues.

You have learned how physical exercise—including aerobic, anaerobic, stretching, and eastern moving meditation techniques (such as tai chi, chi gung, and some of the other "soft" martial arts)—increases body awareness, improves organ and gland function, and boosts the benefits of the meditation/visualization techniques. These latter components of the fibroid-healing program address past traumas that may have created emotional issues. As you know, these issues could be around relationship problems, physical or emotional abuse, unresolved creative concerns, or the inability to eliminate unwanted elements in your life and/or bring in those elements you need for your own self-actualization. Emotional issues create energy stagnation and "armoring" of fascial tissue in the pelvic area that impedes energy flow and can set you up for fibroid tumors.

• Patient and doctor work toward the goal of feeling fully alive, a condition of optimal physical, environmental, mental, emotional, spiritual, and social health.

This principle of holistic health stresses the point that the fibroid-healing program is not limited to easing the symptoms of your condition. It is equally committed to promoting harmony and balance throughout every aspect of your life. In that way, your overall health is addressed and the fibroid condition becomes a vehicle for your personal growth, on all levels. In *Cancer as a Turning Point,* psychotherapist Lawrence Leshan suggests transforming a diagnosis of cancer from a death sentence into a challenge to remake your life. In the same way, your fibroid condition can become an opportunity to reevaluate your life, to see where your life is not as you want it to be and where you can make changes that will promote your balance and development. This program can be your guide in that process toward creating the life you want. The message of your fibroid condition and the healing principles of this program can help you remake any aspects of your life that are not promoting your overall balance and peak health.

• Unconditional love, the final principle of holistic health, may be the most relevant in our increasingly rushed and impersonal world.

Love is the most powerful healer. I am not talking about the "flower power" brand of sex, drugs, and rock & roll free love in the sixties. I am referring to the energy addressed to by all the world's major religions and philosophies—what the Chinese call chi, the Japanese term ki, Hindus refer to as prana, Christians call Christ consciousness, and Jews speak of as chai. My greatest healing lesson has been learning how to cultivate unconditional love. I know that when I am not judging myself—that is, when I am loving myself unconditionally—life is good and everyone who comes into my orbit of influence feels better for it. You have had the experience of being with someone in a down mood and sensing how that person's emotional state can make you either feel down yourself or arouse your urge to get away. On the other hand, when you are in the presence of a person who radiates love and acceptance, your sense of well-being improves. We affect each other in this way because our energies are all interconnected on a deep level. Try this simple test. The next time you are driving, whenever it is safe to do so—say, at a stoplight—look at the driver in the car next to yours and smile. Invariably, that driver will turn and look you right in the eye and smile back at you. After many years of looking away as soon as eye contact is made, I now smile at the other person in acknowledgment of this pleasing human connection that joins us in positive energy and the tacit understanding that it is really good to be alive.

As adults, we have been given an enormous responsibility for the growth and development of our children. The most effective way to teach them is by setting an example of self-nurturing without being selfish.

Now, let us get down to the nuts and bolts of how you can implement all that you have learned.

Getting Started

As Eileen scooped up my typed instructions for the next few months of her personal fibroid-healing program, I observed a look in her eyes that I had seen in other patients many times before. Eileen was overwhelmed by the number of changes she would have to make in her life in order to heal her fibroid. She knew that these changes were necessary, including saying goodbye to many of her favorite foods—standard American diet staples like fast-food hamburgers, pizza, breads, rolls, dairy products, and doughnuts, invariably washed down with diet soft drinks. Eileen's supplement experience had never gone beyond the occasional Price Club multivitamin. It was not surprising that taking the brief list of supplements I had advised seemed like an enormous burden. Yet Eileen was familiar with herbal products and had even taken echinacea once or twice to treat colds. Now, however, the amount of herbal compounds I wanted her to take had become another source of her distress.

Still, Eileen found these aspects of the program daunting but manageable. What really stretched her concept of medical treatment to the breaking point were the daily castor oil packs and accompanying mediation-visualization exercises that involved exploring her past for situations that may have affected her fibroid condition. To Eileen, this was the same as blaming herself for her condition, a way of saying that she had done this to herself. Eileen was aware of treatments like acupuncture and other modalities that work on the body's energetic level, but she was not ready to explore possible emotional issues that may have been associated with her fibroids. Deep down inside, Eileen knew that the meditation–castor-oil-pack sessions would eventually lead her to these issues, because we had already discussed the role of triggering events in fibroid conditions. But she did not want to go there. Concerns over the issue of self-guilt made Eileen reluctant to consider possible connections between her fibroids and buried emotional issues.

I realized that Eileen needed a safe and familiar place in which to begin her program, because she could not jump right into these new and strange healing therapies all at once. I told her that I understood how overwhelming all of this must seem. She responded by admitting that the program was so challenging that she was afraid she might give up and wind up doing nothing. I suggested that Eileen take the material home to read and discuss with her partner. At the end of the week, we would meet again to go over any questions about the program and set up successive steps for implementing the various aspects of the program. We would move slowly, adding new aspects of the program only after Eileen had become accustomed to the previous ones. This plan sounded workable to her. She gave me a relieved smile as she picked up her instructions again and arranged her next appointment.

This slow but steady incremental approach to her fibroid-healing program worked for Eileen. Staying on her program became progressively easier, because with each additional element, she was able to experience increased relief from her fibroid symptoms. After several months, her fibroids stopped growing and she was able to make it to menopause, when the fibroids shrank substantially and were no longer a problem.

Biological Individuality

Eileen's story relates to a key consideration in anyone's healing process, the concept of biological individuality. Developed in the fifties by nutritional biochemist Roger Williams, this concept is based on the truth that we do not live in a one-size-fits-all world, especially when it comes to nutrition and how we interact with our environment. Each of us possesses a set of genes that distinguishes us from anyone else on the planet. In addition, each of us has been exposed to a unique environment that affects the expression of our individual genes in specific ways. This environment includes what we eat, how we exercise, our stressors and how we deal with them, and our personal perspective on the world. For example, do we see the universe as nurturing, with an abundance of energy and resources to meet our needs, or is the universe a threatening and dangerous place in which we constantly need to be on guard? The sum total of your unique genes and individual environment makes up your own biological individuality, and your individuality can express itself in the way in which you respond to a healing program. It determines whether you can jump right into the total package or whether it is better for you to introduce elements of that complex program more gradually, a few at a time.

Some people order all the supplements and put together a schedule for their new diet, vitamin, herb, and hormone regimen right away. They even have put into place a system of eliminating foods in order to determine possible sensitivities, by their second day on the program. They embark on measures to improve intestinal and liver function and even strengthen their adrenal glands with the meditation and visualizations associated with castor oil packs. Perhaps they join a health club, and hire a personal trainer to instruct them on the proper way to get started in their weight training and bodybuilding exercises, and sign up for tai chi classes.

Obviously, not all of you are able to proceed right away with this full-steam-ahead effort and focused determination. Some of you may be so drained and exhausted by your condition that there just is not sufficient energy available to launch a mammoth effort all at once. I have found many people are like Eileen. If they try to start the entire program at once, they feel so overwhelmed that they wind up doing nothing at all, which is why I am telling you what I always tell my patients: pick one aspect of the program that feels possible to accomplish and get started on that one component only. For some of you, beginning to eat differently is a great place to start. Others can start with the exercise, yoga, and meditation practice. Still others may decide to begin the program with some herbs and nutrients that can help restore balance. I have also worked with several women who were so enervated and overwhelmed by their condition that they could not even get out of bed without the help of medication. So, their healing programs began with medications like Prozac, which helped them get through their days and find the energy and will to start the other aspects of their healing. We could eliminate the Prozac when they began to heal.

The effects of biological individuality are as many as there are people on this planet. Some patients tell me that the vitamin and mineral supplements make them nauseous or that they cause other negative gastrointestinal symptoms, such as gas, diarrhea, or constipation. That lets me know these patients first need to do intestinal restoration work before their systems can handle supplements. Their intestinal dysbiosis, or imbalance, and possible leaky gut (caused by an overabundance of the yeast organism known as *Candida albicans,* as well as harmful bacteria and parasites) means that not only will supplements add to their distress, but also these women are not able to absorb important nutrients that they are ingesting in their food. These intestinal problems must be addressed first, before any other components of the healing program are put into place. If not, these patients will not see any signs of improvement in their condition, and they are likely to give up on the program.

If you can imagine the state of your health as a circular maze with optimal health in the center, you will realize that there are many entrances to the maze on the outside and that many paths will take you to that center. (See illustration on p. 258.) We can start our progress toward optimal health from several possible points—from dietary changes to Prozac—and still find our ways to the prize of

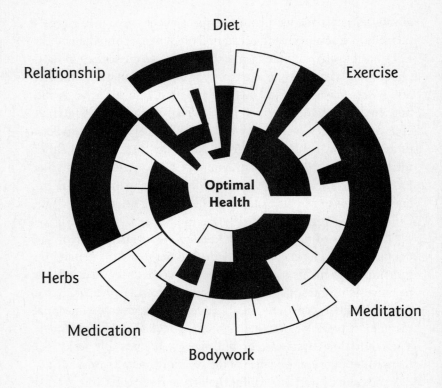

Diet

Relationship

Exercise

Optimal
Health

Herbs

Meditation

Medication

Bodywork

optimal health. Or you can launch your effort from many different entrance points at the same time, and move effectively in that way toward better health.

Working with Your Doctor

None of the natural treatments I have described in this book—including diet, exercise, body-mind work, herbs, and supplements—conflict with each other or with conventional medical fibroid treatments because they work by stimulating your body to regain its balance and energy, and they help enhance your health overall. These healing techniques can only augment the effectiveness of whatever conventional treatments you may also undergo. Even if you do have some type of surgery for your fibroid condition, these health-improving strategies will allow for a more successful outcome and a speedier healing. If your uterus and ovaries are preserved, the healing program addresses whatever energy imbalances triggered the fibroid condition in the first place and will help prevent the fibroids from regrowing.

Partnering with a Health-Care Provider

Three key factors predict the success of any woman's fibroid-healing program:

1. MUTUAL TRUST BETWEEN THE PATIENT AND THE PRACTITIONER. I cannot help thinking in this regard of a recent patient who was especially nervous, anxious, and even angry over her fibroid condition. She was even more disturbed by her experiences with other gynecologists, who all recommended some kind of invasive surgical procedure. Those emotions created a wall that stood between us throughout our one-hour-long consultation. Trust must develop between patient and doctor during that initial visit for subsequent treatment to be successful. No matter what I tried, I could not get through to this patient. In the end, I was unable to help her because I could not win her trust.

2. THE COMMITMENT AND AWARENESS OF BOTH PATIENT AND THE PRACTITIONER.

3. SUFFICIENT TIME FOR THE PROGRAM TO WORK. If the fibroid condition constitutes an emergency, there may not be enough time for the program to address the condition and reverse its course. If you recall, almost all women who undergo surgery for fibroids are "forced" into the operating room by abnormal vaginal bleeding, pain, and pressure. The nonsurgical, natural treatments that can alleviate those symptoms and render surgery unnecessary require time to do their job.

In the case of the distrustful patient, subsequent visits could have broken down her wall and established our relationship, but her serious fibroid condition simply did not allow enough time.

The relationship built on trust and honesty that exists between doctor and patient is like a third entity, and it is a key component in healing. The more experience I gain from working with patients, the more I view myself as a facilitator for other people's inner healers. I believe that each of us possesses an inherent ability to heal ourselves. It is just that most of us have forgotten how. I am not even sure exactly how this healing happens. I do know, though, that when a person brings as much of his, or her, life as possible into physical, emotional, and spiritual balance, an energy state of optimal well-being is created in which the life-force can flow freely. It may actually be as simple as the fact that we are energetic beings and the more closely we harmonize with the energy of the universe, the healthier we become.

I am not saying that you must have blind, uncritical faith in your doctors. The information you gain from this book will better prepare you to evaluate the possible effectiveness of any doctor you may choose to visit. Once you have established that you do want to work with this person, try to be open and positive about your medical outcome. Work with him or her as an active partner in your own healing, and do not be afraid to make your own suggestions when creating your healing program.

Here are a few tips that will help you prepare for a visit to the doctor or any other health-care practitioner:

• Bring in a written list of what you want to accomplish during this particular visit and go over the list during the first part of your interview. One of the most frustrating situations for both myself and for a patient is for her to say at the very end of her visit, after her healing program has been set up, "Oh doctor, I forgot to say. What do you think this pain is that I've been having?" It could be that this pain could be dealt with during a subsequent visit, but it may also have some bearing on the present condition and should have been factored in when I was creating her healing program.

• Bring with you all relevant lab work, including sonograms, MRIs, CAT scans, and other X-ray results. Most gynecologists do not read X-rays themselves, but they will be interested in seeing the reports on those tests. Other gynecologists, like myself, prefer to do their own sonograms at the time of the exam. This is important because I can use sonograms during the exam to teach the patient a great deal about her fibroids, as well as about normal and abnormal pelvic anatomy. This will also enhance the effectiveness of the patient's visualization–castor-oil-pack sessions, because once she sees her own anatomy, she can more readily visualize it. I also find that doing my own sonograms in real time gives me much more information than just viewing someone else's pictures and reading their report.

• Bring all current and relevant blood and saliva tests and a list of all the medications and supplements you are taking.

Health Is a State of Balance

I have described optimal health as a state of balance. You may be wondering how you can tell when you are out of balance, other than by the fact of your fibroid condition. Believe me, when we are out of balance, we know it. All the aspects of our lives that we took for granted—sleep patterns, energy levels, sexual desire, and relatively even moods—seem to deteriorate. You become afflicted with more and more mysterious aches and pains. You may even greet each new day with a headache. Shall I go on?

Once we recognize that we are out of balance, what is the next step? I believe that the next step is recognizing the need to make some changes and being willing to do so. I am constantly amazed and impressed by the amount of research some patients bring to my office, even on their first visits. In fact, my patients often have brought new facts or ideas to my attention that I needed to explore further. The healing programs I develop for individual patients are based on many different healing modalities, and I have discovered some of these techniques through my patients' research. All these women gathered their information because they were aware of some imbalance that was affecting their health. They desired to address that imbalance and make whatever changes would help them do so. Each had invested valuable time and energy to help herself discover what needed to change and how to do it.

Part of that process of change often means finding a holistic health-care provider who is willing listen to you and view you as his or her partner in the process of finding the right path to your healing.

Is There Enough Time?

The final consideration in your fibroid-healing program is: does your condition allow you enough time to effect a change, or is the state of your fibroids at a point where you will soon be forced to use an invasive procedure? The symptoms that are most difficult to gauge are heavy bleeding and severe pain. As I have mentioned already, hemorrhagic-type bleeding is the most likely reason for an invasive procedure. If your condition allows enough time for correcting whatever imbalances are associated with the bleeding, then surgery can be avoided. But if the condition is too far advanced and excessive bleeding continues unabated, the program will not eliminate the need for surgery. In some cases, though, surgery can be avoided if the healing program receives an extra boost from another therapy, such as acupuncture and traditional Chinese medicine.

Cindy was slim and fit and followed a health-promoting lifestyle. But this forty-year-old was plagued with the symptoms of subserous and intramural fibroids. She had long ago given up on conventional medical help because every doctor she saw told her that her condition eventually would bring her to the operating room. Cindy consulted many holistic doctors and tried many different treatments. First, there were herbalists, then a homeopath. She even had undergone a course of acupuncture treatments. At first, each of these techniques seemed to work. Then, all too soon, the clotting and cramping of her periods invariably returned. Now, the small fibroids she had known about for a long time seemed to be growing. Each of the healing modalities she tried is both a healing science and holistic art, but, for some reason, Cindy was not responding. When she consulted with me, I put Cindy on a comprehensive fibroid-healing program, and she stuck to it faithfully. But the results were just as dismal: short-term relief, followed by the return of all her symptoms. I realized that some other element was missing in this effort to return her to balance. If we did not put it into place soon, she was headed for the operating room. It was only after Cindy had the idea of adding regular acupuncture sessions to her fibroid-healing program that she finally shrank her fibroids, was relieved of their symptoms, and achieved lasting healing.

ACUPUNCTURE

Many of my patients also consult experts in Eastern medical modalities, such as acupuncture, to further strengthen and heal by stimulating the body's own healing powers. Acupuncture is growing more popular by the day, and many conventional medical doctors are incorporating this technique and other ancient healing systems into their practices. Acupuncture schools are opening up all over the country, and licensing boards have been set up in most states to regulate practitioners and protect clients.

An acupuncturist promotes balance and healing by locating energy blockages and inserting fine needles into specific points to free blockages and restore proper energy flow and health. Western bodywork and therapeutic touch therapies that stem from these eastern practices, such as rolfing and the Alexander Technique, also aim to prevent health problems—particularly those inhibiting full pelvic function—by strengthening and balancing the patient, physically and mentally.

I encourage you to be as proactive as Cindy and many of my

other patients and to view your fibroid condition as a challenge to grow, to become more informed, and to take charge of your own health. Once you are able to drop the mentality of a victim searching for a rescuer, you will find that everything around you shifts. You will find the right health-care provider, the right information, and possibly even a community of other women with fibroids with whom you can share information and support. Actually, the fact that you are now reading this final page of *Healing Fibroids* means you are already on your way to better health and healing.

RESOURCE GUIDE

Vegetarian Cookbooks

Behnke, Allison, ed. *Vegetarian Cooking Around the World*. Minneapolis: Lerner Publishing Group, 2002.

Fetterly, Mary-Jo. *The "I Can't Believe It's Vegetarian" Cookbook*. Mary-Jo Fetterly, 2000.

Shaw, Diana. *The Essential Vegetarian Cookbook: Your Guide to the Best Foods on Earth*. New York: Clarkson Potter, 1997.

Sperling, Virginia, and Christine McFadden. *The Complete Book of Vegetarian Cooking*. Smithmark Publishing, 1996.

Note: Lerner Publications has put out a series of *Easy Menu Cookbooks* covering virtually every ethnic cuisine. Each includes vegetarian recipes. Example: Rose Coronado, *Cooking the Mexican Way: Revised and Expanded to Include New Low-Fat and Vegetarian Recipes*.

Books on Natural Healing

Appleton, Nancy. *Lick the Sugar Habit*. New York: Avery Penguin Putnam, 1996.

Atkins, Robert C. *Dr. Atkins' Health Revolution: How Complementary Medicine Can Extend Your Life*. New York: Bantam, 1990.

Bailey, Covert. *The New Fit or Fat*. New York: Houghton Mifflin, 1991.

Baker, Sidney MacDonald. *Detoxification & Healing: The Key to Optimal Health*. New York: Keats, 1997.

Barnes, Broda, and Lawrence Galton. *Hypothyroidism: The Unsuspected Illness*. New York: Ty Crowell Co., 1976.

Bechtel, Stefan. *The Practical Encyclopedia of Sex and Health: From Aphrodisiacs and Hormones to Potency, Stress, Vasectomy and Yeast Infections*. Emmaus, Pa.: Rodale Press, 1993.

Benson, Herbert. *The Relaxation Response*. New York: Avon, 1990.

————. *Timeless Healing*. New York: Fireside, Simon & Schuster, 1997.

Bland, Jeffrey, with Sara Benum. *The 20-Day Rejuvenation Diet Program*. New York: Keats, 1996.

Brody, Jane. *Jane Brody's Guide to Personal Health*. New York: Avon, 1982.

Bry, Adelaide, with Marjorie Bair. *Directing the Movies of Your Mind: Visualization for Health and Insight*. New York: Harper & Row, 1978.

Carson, Rachel. *Silent Spring*. New York: Houghton Mifflin, 1999.

Chan, Pedro. *Finger Acupressure*. New York: Ballantine, 1975.

Chia, Mantak. *Healing Love Through the Tao: Cultivating Female Sexual Energy*. Huntington, N.Y.: Healing Tao Books, 1986.

Childre, Doc Lew. *Freeze-Frame*. Boulder Creek, Calif.: Planetary, 1994.

Colbin, Annemarie. *Food and Healing*. New York: Ballantine, 1986.

Cousens, Gabriel. *Conscious Eating*. Berkeley, Calif.: North Atlantic, 2000.

Csikszentmihalyi, Mihaly. *Flow: The Psychology of Optimal Experience*. New York: Harper & Row, 1990.

D'Adamo, Peter J. *Eat Right for Your Type*. New York: Putnam, 1996.

DeCava, Judith A. *The Real Truth about Vitamins and Antioxidants*. Columbus, Ga.: Brentwood Academic Press, 1996.

Dossey, Larry. *Healing Words*. New York: HarperCollins, 1993.

————. *Prayer Is Good Medicine.* New York: HarperCollins, 1996.

Elias, Jason, and Shelagh Ryan Masline. *The A to Z Guide to Healing Herbal Remedies.* New York: Dell, 1995.

Epstein, Gerald. *Healing Visualizations: Creating Health Through Imagery.* New York: Bantam, 1989.

Erasmus, Udo. *Fats That Heal, Fats That Kill.* Burnaby, BC, Canada: Alive Books, 1993.

Gach, Michael Reed. *Acupressure's Potent Points: A Guide to Self-Care for Common Ailments.* New York: Bantam, 1990.

Galland, Leo. *Power Healing: Use the New Integrated Medicine to Cure Yourself.* New York: Random House, 1997.

Gladstar, Rosemary. *Herbal Healing for Women.* New York: Fireside, Simon & Schuster, 1993.

Golan, Ralph. *Optimal Wellness.* New York: Ballantine, 1995.

Goldfarb, Herbert A., M.D., with Judith Grief. *The No-Hysterectomy Option: Your Body—Your Choice.* New York: John Wiley & Sons, 1990.

Goleman, Daniel, and Joel Gurin, eds. *Mind Body Medicine: How to Use Your Mind for Better Health.* Yonkers, N.Y.: Consumer Reports Books, 1995.

Haich, Elisabeth. *Sexual Energy and Yoga.* Santa Fe: Aurora Press, 1983.

Hay, Louise L. *Heal Your Body.* Carlsbad, Calif.: Hay House, 1994.

Hobbs, Christopher. *Women's Herbs, Women's Health.* Loveland, Colo.: Interweave Press, 1998.

Hoffman, David. *The New Holistic Herbal.* Boston: Element, 1983.

Kabat-Zinn, Jon. *Full Catastrophe Living: Using the Wisdom of Your Body and Mind to Face Stress-Related Illness.* New York: Delta, 1990.

Keck, Robert. *Sacred Quest.* West Chester, Pa.: Chrysalis, 2000.

Kloss, Jethro. *Back to Eden.* Santa Barbara: Woodbridge Press, 1983.

Kordel, Lelord. *Natural Folk Remedies.* New York: Putnam, 1974.

Lark, Susan M. *Fibroid Tumors & Endometriosis.* Berkeley, Calif.: Celestial Arts, 1993.

Lee, John. *What Your Doctor May Not Tell You About Premenopause*. New York: Warner Books, 1999.

Levine, Barbara Hoberman. *Your Body Believes Every Word You Say*. Fairfield, Conn.: Aslan, 1991.

Lowen, Alexander. *The Betrayal of the Body*. New York: Collier, 1967.

Lozoff, Bo. *It's a Meaningful Life*. New York: Viking Penguin, 2000.

Masline, Shelagh Ryan, and Barbara Close. *Aromatherapy: The A–Z Guide to Healing with Essential Oils*. New York: Dell, 1998.

Mendelsohn, Robert S. *Male Practice: How Doctors Manipulate Women*. Lincolnwood, Fla.: Contemporary, 1981.

Mindell, Earl. *Earl Mindell's Vitamin Bible*. New York: Warner, 1991.

Moses, Marion. *Designer Poisons: How to Protect Your Health and Home from Toxic Pesticides*. San Francisco: The Pesticide Education Center, 1995.

Murray, Michael T. *The Healing Power of Herbs: The Enlightened Person's Guide to the Wonders of Medicinal Plants*. Rocklin, Calif.: Prima, 1995.

Myss, Caroline. *Why People Don't Heal*. New York: Three Rivers, 1998.

———, and C. Norman Shealy. *Anatomy of the Spirit*. New York: Random House, 1997.

Nelson, Miriam. *Strong Women Stay Young*. New York: Bantam, 1998.

Nissim, Rina. *Natural Healing in Gynecology*. London: Pandora, 1986.

Northrup, Christiane. *Women's Bodies, Women's Wisdom*. New York: Bantam, 1995.

Ohashi, Wataru. *Do-It-Yourself Shiatsu*. New York: Dutton, 1976.

Oki, Mashahito. *Zen Yoga Therapy*. Tokyo: Japan Books, 1979.

Oumano, Elena. *A Handbook of Natural Folk Remedies*. New York: Avon, 1997.

———. *Natural Sex*. New York: Dutton/Plume, 1999.

Parvati, Jeanne. *Herbs & Things: Jeanne Rose's Herbal.* New York: Workman, 1972.

Pearl, Bill. *Getting Stronger.* New York: Random House, 1996.

Pelletier, Kenneth R. *Mind as Healer, Mind as Slayer: A Holistic Approach to Preventing Stress Disorder.* New York: Delta, 1977.

Pert, Candace. *Molecules of Emotion.* New York: Scribner, 1997.

Phillips, David A. *Guidebook to Nutritional Factors in Foods.* Santa Barbara: Woodbridge Press, 1979.

Pizzorno, Joseph. *Total Wellness.* Rocklin, Calif.: Prima, 1996.

Robbins, John. *Diet for a New America.* Tiburon, Calif.: H. J. Kramer, 1987.

————. *Reclaiming Our Health.* Tiburon, Calif.: H. J. Kramer, 1996.

Salaman, Maureen, with James F. Scheer. *Foods That Heal.* Menlo Park, Calif.: Statford, 1989.

Schmidt, Michael. *Smart Fats.* Berkeley, Calif.: Frog, 1997.

Scott, Julian, and Susan Scott. *Natural Medicine for Women.* New York: Gaia Books, 1991.

Selye, Hans. *Stress Without Distress.* New York: Signet, 1974.

Siegel, Bernie. *Love, Medicine & Miracles.* New York: HarperPerennial, 1990.

Skilling, Johanna. *Fibroids: The Complete Guide to Taking Charge of Your Physical, Emotional, and Spiritual Well-Being.* New York: Marlowe and Co., 2000.

Steinman, David, and R. Michael Wisner. *Living Healthy in a Toxic World.* New York: Berkley Publishing Group, 1996.

Tierra, Michael. *The Way of Herbs.* New York: Washington Square Press, 1983.

Tyler, Varro E., and Steven Foster. *Tyler's Honest Herbal.* Binghamton, N.Y.: The Haworth Press, 1999.

Weed, Susun S. *Wise Woman Herbal for the Childbearing Year.* Woodstock, N.Y.: Ash Tree, 1985.

White, Bowen F. *Why Normal Isn't Healthy.* City Center, Minn.: Hazelden, 2000.

Yetiv, Jack Z. *Popular Nutritional Practices: Sense and Nonsense.* New York: Dell, 1988.

Zukav, Gary. *The Seat of the Soul.* New York: Fireside, Simon & Schuster, 1990.

Mail Order Companies

FOR ORGANIC FOODS, SUPPLEMENTS, AND HERBAL REMEDIES . . .

Lifethyme store: 212-420-9099

Hickey Chemists: 800-724-5566

L&H Vitamins: 800-221-1152

Vitamin Direct: 800-468-4027

Freeda Vitamins: 800-777-3737

Needs: 800-634-1380

AmeriHerb, Inc.: 800-267-6141

A Catalogue of Herbal Delights: 800-879-3337

Abundant Life Herbal Supply: 510-939-7857

Vitamin Trader: 800-334-9300

Phillips Nutritionals: 800-582-8461

Vitamin Discount Connection: 888-848-2110

The Vitamin Zone: 800-583-1187

The Vitamin Shoppe: 800-223-1216

Phyto Pharmacia: 800-553-2370

Metagenics: 800-638-2848

Gaia Herbs: gaiaherbs.com

Emerson Ecologics (for vitamins and other nutraceuticals, including castor oil packs): 800-654-4432

FOR ORGANIC FOODS, NATURAL CLEANSERS, CLOTHING, AND LINEN . . .

Harmony Products: 800-869-3446

Self Care: 800-345-3371

Natural Lifestyle Supplies: 800-752-2775

The Allergy Store: 800-824-7163
Bollinger Fitness Equipment: www.bollingerfitness.com
Natural Products: www.realgoods.com

Recommended Magazines:

Natural Health: 800-526-8440
New Age: 800-782-7006
Yoga Journal: 800-436-9642
Alternative Medicine Digest: 800/415-435-1779

To Find a Holistic Physician:

American Holistic Medical Association: 703-556-9245
American Board of Holistic Medicine: 425-741-2996

To Have Your 2-OH and 16 Alpha OH Estrogen Ratio Measured:

Great Smokies Diagnostic Lab: www.gsdl.com
Metametrix Lab: 800-221-4640

INDEX

* Page numbers for illustrations are italicized.